mostly straight

mostly straight

sexual fluidity among men

RITCH C. SAVIN-WILLIAMS

**Cuyahoga Falls
Library**
Cuyahoga Falls, Ohio

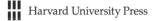 Harvard University Press

CAMBRIDGE, MASSACHUSETTS ≈ LONDON, ENGLAND 2017

First printing

Library of Congress Cataloging-in-Publication Data

Names: Savin-Williams, Ritch C., author.
Title: Mostly straight : sexual fluidity among men / Ritch C. Savin-Williams.
Description: Cambridge, Massachusetts : Harvard University Press, 2017. |
    Includes bibliographical references and index.
Identifiers: LCCN 2017018927 | ISBN 9780674976382 (alk. paper)
Subjects: LCSH: Young bisexual men—Interviews. | Sexual minorities. | Sex. |
    Sex role. | Sex (Psychology) | Sex (Biology)
Classification: LCC HQ74.7 .S38 2017 | DDC 306.76—dc23
LC record available at https://lccn.loc.gov/2017018927

contents

preface

[I've never been] opposed to gay interactions. I've joked about it with my friends. I got close once but never made out, though we are physical.

(DILLON, AGE 20)

IF YOU'RE STRAIGHT, YOUNG, AND MALE and have or believe you might have a slight degree of sexual or romantic attraction to other guys, this book is for you. If you'd like to know more or if these feelings mystify you such that you want to figure out what is going on, this book is for you. If you're a girlfriend, a friend, a sibling, or a parent and you've wondered whether your boyfriend, friend, brother, or son might be "a little bit gay," this book is also for you. Or if you're simply intrigued and want to know about the life experiences of this particular group of young male millennials, read on.

In this book, you'll meet forty young men who are mostly straight. You'll hear their life stories, and perhaps something they say or have done or have come to understand about themselves might resonate with you or someone you know. A mostly straight young person can feel alone or weird, and hearing from other mostly straight young men may help him lead his own distinctive, self-fulfilling life. If you are not mostly straight, then my intention is to help you understand and, I hope, celebrate these young men as they navigate their sexual and romantic lives in an increasingly complicated world.

What we know is that the mostly straight male is the new kid on the block. We hear a lot about the Big Three Sexualities— straight, bisexual, and gay. Most of us assume that these three orientations encompass the universe of sexual identities. If we are prepared to accept mostly straight as a fourth sexual identity, we gain an increasingly nuanced understanding of sexual orientation—and its close cousin, romantic orientation. We won't stop at four; no doubt we will soon recognize additional sexual identities.

To the uninitiated, "mostly straight" may seem paradoxical. How can a man be *mostly* heterosexual? Women, we know, can be sexually fluid, as the sizable literature on the subject attests. But if you're a young man, you might assume that either you're straight or you're not, meaning you're bisexual or gay. Yet mostly straight men exist. In fact, the evidence suggests that more young men identify or describe themselves as mostly straight than identify as either bisexual or gay combined.

In the most general sense, a mostly straight young man is *sexually* and / or *romantically distinctive;* we might say that he's *fluid* or *flexible,* supposedly an alien feature of male sexuality. Traditionally, our understanding has been that if you're male and have even a slight attraction to the same sex, then you must be bisexual or gay. Even if this isn't immediately apparent, it will become so once you come to terms with your true self and exit your "phase" of bicuriosity or questioning. Women, by contrast, can be mostly straight because they are less constrained than men by culturally strict gender and sexual norms. This kind of thinking dictates that the only options for men are straight, bisexual, or gay, not *something else.* If you're a mostly straight young man, you know these assumptions are wrong, and you're not alone.

A recent U.S. government poll found that among 18- to 24-year-old men, 6 percent marked their sexual attractions as "mostly opposite sex." That's more than fifteen million young men. Yet when these men were forced to choose either straight or bisexual as a sexual identity, about three-quarters marked straight because for them bisexual, even if it is understood as "bisexual-leaning straight," is too gay to accurately describe their identity. Given such constraints, these young men were left with no place to truthfully register their sexuality, thus forcing them to be less than honest.

The category "mostly straight" is a recent addition that was not readily available to previous generations of men. A new survey revealed striking contrasts across age groups. One question asked, "Thinking about sexuality, which of the following comes closer to your view?"

- "There is no middle ground—you are either heterosexual or you are not."
- "Sexuality is a scale—it is possible to be somewhere near the middle."

A majority of millennials endorsed the second option, which means they believe in a spectrum of sexuality. Adults from other generations preferred the first, which signifies a two-category approach—straight, not straight—to sexuality.

Millennials were also less likely than other groups to label themselves as "completely heterosexual." And even among those who identified as straight, they were more likely than their parents' generation to respond to the following three questions with "Very unlikely, but not impossible" or "Maybe, if I really liked them." The lead-in was, "If the right person came along at the right time . . ."

- "Do you think it is conceivable that you could be attracted to a person of the same sex?"
- "Do you think it is conceivable that you could have a sexual experience with a person of the same sex?"
- "Do you think it is conceivable that you could have a relationship with a person of the same sex?"

To each of these questions, their parents' generation overwhelmingly responded with "Absolutely not."

Identifying as mostly straight is now largely possible because the millennial generation is adding new complexity to sexual and romantic relationships. Over the last several years the Pew Research Center has reported on the characteristics of millennials.

The *New York Times* branded the cohort as "Generation Nice." What does *nice* mean? Contrasted with previous generations, young people today are more confident, connected, introspective, and open to change. They're skeptical of traditional institutions and ways of viewing the world, and they are willing to improvise solutions that are both creative and good for the environment and future generations. As adolescents and young adults, they are happier and more satisfied with their lives than previous generations. They express liberal, progressive attitudes toward religion and race relations, social policies, and sexuality.

How do these values and practices play out in the sexual and romantic lives of mostly straights? In the following pages, I'll introduce you to mostly straight young men as they tell their life stories. The first thing you'll notice is that they're a very diverse group. In high school, they were hipsters, jocks, nerds, druggies, skaters, class clowns, burnouts, and straight-laced achievers. Long hair, short hair, clean-shaven, bearded, tattooed, pierced, muscular, lanky, hyper, and pudgy. They want to change the world, fit in, drop out, go into medicine, advocate marketing strategies, fight for social justice, write novels, or be unemployed, and many have no clue what they'll do.

You will first meet Josh Hutcherson and several other media stars who are neither straight nor gay but mostly straight. Then comes Dillon, a young man whose story lies at the heart of this book. It might seem inconceivable that Dillon, a hockey goalie in college who loved frat parties and said he intended to have lots of casual sex with young women during his college years, identifies as anything other than totally, exclusively straight. How could he be *mostly* straight?

Dillon and others, including Kyle, Carlos, Demetri, Ryan, and Luke, will tell you about their sexual and romantic development from their first sexual memory, their first crush, their first orgasm, their first sex, and their first true love. Finally, they'll speculate about what being mostly straight means for their sexual and romantic future—which might be yours as well if you are a mostly straight young man.

mostly straight

the sexual neverlands

*If the guy is attractive enough . . .
You just never know.* (DILLON, AGE 20)

MANY OF YOU might find yourselves in a place Dillon called the *sexual neverlands,* a region between heterosexuality and bisexuality without a name or an identity—until now. In previous generations, a youth might have called himself "straight but not narrow," "heteroflexible," "bending a little," "bicurious," or, as one young man claimed, "a dude, most of the time." Or perhaps you have your own description that best reflects this undiscovered country where your sexual and romantic lives reside.

Now, this *dude* has a home, an identity that makes sense to him and is gaining widespread acceptance. He's *mostly straight.* He belongs to a growing trend of young men who are secure in their heterosexuality yet remain aware of their potential to experience far more. Perhaps he's felt attracted to or fantasized about another guy to a slight degree or intermittently. He might or might not be comfortable with this seeming contradiction, a hetero guy who, despite his lust for women, rejects a straight label, a sexual category, and a sexual description that feels foreign. He'd rather find another place on the sexual/romantic continuum, some location that fits him more comfortably.

More specifically, the dilemma is how best to define such a young man. He knows he's not gay, but straight with a dash of gayness. But how much gayness? Not much—a relatively small percentage, say around 5 percent to 10 percent, of his sexual and romantic feelings. Strict rules don't apply. These attractions are sexual, romantic, or both and can be expressed in various ways, from erotic fantasies to actual behavior. Perhaps he's made out or he wants to make out with a guy friend. He's participated in a group jerk-off or is willing to receive oral sex from an attractive guy he's just met. But it's unlikely that he has had actual sex with a guy, though he might be willing to if the right guy or circumstance appeared. He might have had an intense guy crush. But to fall passionately in love with a guy is too much, though he might have quite strong feelings and cuddle with a best friend.

He feels his same-sex sexuality *internally* more than he lives it *externally*. Perhaps if his culture were not so stigmatizing of same-sex sexuality he might be more inclined to express himself through tangible expressions of sex or romance—not frequently but occasionally. Because many in his generation have forcefully rejected the idea that some sexualities are more valuable than others, he might still have a chance to communicate the complexity of his sexuality and romantic desires in ways that feel comfortable to him and transparent to you, even if you're not mostly straight yourself.

Developmentally, this slight degree of gayness has probably been present since birth or before, though we really don't know because no one has ever explored the origins of *mostly heterosexuality*. Is it an orientation point along a continuum, just to the right of heterosexuality? Or is it inhabited by straight guys who want to give the impression that they are progressive in their sexuality? Is it a matter of sexuality or of personality traits? Perhaps the pool of straight guys with same-sex attractions is large, but only those with personality characteristics such as curiosity, impulsiveness, sensation seeking, sexual excitability, and sexual openness become mostly straight. These traits might motivate such young men to seek the full range of their sexual or romantic desires, or they might become aroused by such longings.

Absent these traits, straight men are not sufficiently intrigued to explore their same-sex romantic or sexual cravings—that is, if they have them. Even though their millennial world now renders same-sex sexuality less of a "big deal," they might well not feel the burn. However, on the optimistic side, with this seismic generational shift, straight youth are more willing to consider fluidity and, if so, to be less afraid to report it because their fear of negative societal consequences is minimal.

In my interviews with mostly straight young men, I heard stories that could support either an orientation or a personality perspective. Being mostly straight was evident in their first memories. That said, few mostly straight youth were willing to engage these issues during their early childhood play, their peer interactions in middle childhood, their initial sexual activities and romantic crushes in late childhood and early adolescence, or their adolescent sexual and romantic relationships. They simply didn't understand that these mixed feelings were unusual. They often assumed that all boys had the same emotions and did the same things.

A boy's awareness of his difference from totally straight boys usually emerges or solidifies with the onset of puberty—which doesn't mean he has a name for it or thinks of it as remarkable or bizarre. Maybe he just feels slightly different without knowing how or why. It likely doesn't intimidate him but intrigues him. Blind about what is going on, he might easily dismiss it, especially if he plays on athletic teams, attends boarding school, belongs to a gang, joins a fraternity, or participates in any other venue where boys exclusively congregate. The extreme devotion boys have for each other appears to all concerned as normal—not a boy crush, but two buds. If the two connect sexually, it's only for pleasure, kept secret, and not talked about. These teens might well be mostly straight—not all, but some. Other boys who don't have these homoerotic experiences but wish they had might also identify as mostly straight.

The emergence of these same-sex attractions has likely been subtle. Usually, it is only late in high school or as a young adult that he can finally assign a name to what he feels. It helps that millennial culture, especially through social media, is increasingly giving notice to sexual and romantic complexity, providing the mostly straight option exposure and a name that decreases its mysterious qualities.

However, adults might not get it, and they may excuse or ignore the behavior of their son, brother, grandson, nephew, or cousin. Some may say, "boys will be boys." More likely, they won't know or particularly care because they unquestionably see the heterosexual side of his life—he's dating girls, and perhaps he's sexually engaging girls. What I object to most strenuously is disparaging mostly heterosexuality as merely an adolescent phenomenon that is outgrown once young adulthood emerges. Sizable numbers of mostly straight youths maintain their mostly straight status not just during adolescence and young adulthood but throughout adulthood, even as they marry or have children.

What do I mean by *sizable numbers?* It's difficult to establish a precise number, but at least half keep their mostly straight identity and likely more. I designed a study to help determine what happens to mostly straight young men over time. I first interviewed them when they were about 20 years old (Time 1) and then contacted them eighteen months later (Time 2). Half of those who were mostly straight at Time 1 stayed that way, and the other half at Time 2 identified as exclusively straight. Their small *drop of gayness* did not propel them any farther toward the gay end of the sexual continuum. None became bisexual or gay. Those who joined the ranks of the mostly straight at Time 2 were previously straight at Time 1. I might add that a few of the young men who now identify as straight are not totally straight; they reported having a small degree of same-sex sexuality. I give them their own chapter, referring to them as *primarily straight* or as they frequently called themselves, *straight, but not totally straight.* Perhaps they represent a fifth sexual orientation between straight and mostly straight. You'll be the judge.

After talking with the forty young men featured in this book, it is my distinct impression that they are not trying to become or move toward something else in their sexual identity. They're not transitioning toward identifying as bisexual or gay. They're not closeted gay men who fear being gay yet want to keep a slight, perhaps secretive, gay side by dangling their potential for guy sex. They're not saying, "I'm available for guys who want to have sex with a straight guy" while enjoying the privileges afforded to heterosexual men in our society. They're not equal opportunity bisexuals in disguise trying to hold out hope for straightness, nor are they afraid to identify as bisexual because of societal stigma and prejudice. They are not disgruntled straight men tired of sex with women, nor are they necessarily unhappy or frustrated with the availability of heterosexual sex.

With the words *mostly straight,* the young men describe a unique sexual identity. If they have second thoughts about their sexuality, they may retreat from a full identification with heterosexuality, but rarely do they gravitate toward bisexuality, and almost never do they move toward homosexuality of any sort. Thus, they are closer cousins to straight guys than to traditional bisexual guys.

Alternatively, you might suspect a mostly straight youth is in reality straight but

- is unhappy with such a label because he desires personal flexibility;
- resists being placed in a rigid sexual identity box;
- loves the person, not the gender (pansexual);
- is queer with a distinct radical political ideology and wants to identify with sexual-minority communities as a comrade;
- enjoys the attention of other males, for whatever psychological reason, and by claiming a little bit of same-sex sexuality he receives what he desires.

These might be true for some young men, to a limited extent, but—as we'll see—those explanations don't apply to the vast majority of mostly straight young men.

The question before us remains: Why would a young man choose the mostly straight option when friends, parents, and the media offer the more readily identifiable and acceptable label of straight? More to the point, who forsakes the straight and goes for the mostly straight? I'm not certain because we don't often ask these kinds of questions and thus we overlook or disregard those who don't fit into an existing sexual category. We like our sexualities simple, especially among our male youths, and we prefer to ignore undue complexity. But then, what to do with the guys we can't understand—the outliers, the quirky individuals who are not easily pigeonholed into a well-delineated identity box?

To the uninitiated, as most of us are, a mostly straight guy is an oxymoron. It fractures the heterosexual agenda—or do we call it a heterosexual lifestyle? If a guy is not *exclusively* into girls, he can't be straight. Doesn't everyone have to pick a side? Yet he hasn't. If a guy says he's straight but falls in love with a guy or becomes erect when fantasizing about a guy, what the hell is he? With the words *mostly straight,* he's describing a unique sexual and romantic identity while maintaining a kinship with his straight brothers. He's in, as Dillon told me, the *sexual neverlands.*

straight but not narrow

But I think defining yourself as 100 percent anything is kind of near-sighted and close-minded. (JOSH HUTCHERSON, AGE 24)

A GUY MIGHT NOT BE TOTALLY STRAIGHT, but no one would know unless he told people or shared it on social media. But some mostly straight men are out and proud. In this chapter we'll meet the actor Josh Hutcherson, star of the *Hunger Games* movie franchise, and in the next chapter Dillon, a goalie for a Division 1 college hockey powerhouse. What they have in common is not only their sexual identity but also their youthfulness and attractiveness. They are both self-aware individuals who are also skeptical that all guys are straight, bisexual, or gay.

Josh Hutcherson cofounded and helped fund the online group Straight But Not Narrow, http://www.straightbutnotnarrow.org (see his video "Josh Hutcherson Is Straight but Not Narrow," at https://www.youtube.com/watch?v=HNqKmdNo8tE). Its purpose is to build and support a team of straight allies for lesbian, gay, bisexual, transgender, and queer communities. Josh told the gay magazine *Out*, "I would probably list myself as mostly straight." He elaborated:

Maybe I could say right now I'm 100 percent straight. But who knows? In a fucking year, I could meet a guy and be like, "Whoa, I'm attracted to this person . . ."

I've met guys all the time that I'm like, Damn, that's a good-looking guy, you know. I've never been, like, Oh, I want to kiss that guy. I really love women. But I think defining yourself as 100 percent anything is kind of near-sighted and close-minded.

In his progressive spirit Josh is typical of his millennial generation. He embraces, in his words, "ambiguity over neat and secure boxes," and this speaks to his bravery and self-confidence. Josh is not afraid to be an open ally to lesbian, gay, bisexual, and transgender (LGBT) communities, especially youth-oriented organizations such as gay-straight alliances in middle and high schools, gay youths growing up in rural areas, and the Trevor Project to stop bullying based on sexuality (gay/lesbian youth) and gender expression (trans youth). His many accolades, such as from the MTV Movie Awards, Teen Choice Awards, and the People's Choice Awards, signal his popularity with young fans.

Other young celebrities have also questioned traditional categories of sexual identity. Consider actor and musician Ezra Miller, age 24, who describes himself as "queer." He says, "The way I would choose to identify myself wouldn't be gay. I've been attracted mostly to 'shes,' but I've been with many people, and I'm open to love wherever it can be." He doesn't call himself mostly straight, but he might well qualify.

Ezra is horrified at the way youths who are not straight are treated. He told the *Daily Beast* and *The Advocate* several years ago, "I think a lot of people are projecting their own troubles and fears concerning sexuality onto those around them . . . It really hurts and divides us all, and in the end, so much of the human experience is shared, so we only end up hating and fearing our own damn selves."

British actor Freddie Fox, age 27, has also embraced the idea that sexuality is on a spectrum. Early in 2015 he told the British newspaper *The Telegraph*, "Most of my life to date has been as a straight man, but who knows what will happen next?"

Freddie refuses to align himself with any specific sexual label because he appreciates both sexes:

> I hope I am the type of person who would fall in love with a person, as opposed to a sex. I've had girlfriends, but I wouldn't wish to say "I am this or I am that," because at some time in my life I might fall in love with a man. I hope that I am the type of person who would fall in love with another person, as opposed to a sex . . . It sounds evasive, but I don't think you can necessarily say you're one thing or another until you're 100 years old and you've done it all . . .
>
> Appreciation of both sexes is actually not new; it's incredibly old, it's Roman, it's Greek, and it is something people can do throughout an entire lifetime, having hugely meaningful relationships, no matter what sex they are.

Similarly, the actor Jack Falahee, age 27, described his sexuality in romantic terms: "I hope I am the type of person who would fall in love with a person, as opposed to a sex."

Jake Uitti, age 33, plays in the band The Great Um and has recently reflected on his life and what he might have missed because of his traditional upbringing:

> I've never really explored my sexuality . . . But I've never pushed myself to determine where my boundaries lie. I've never felt attracted to men, for example, but I've also always wondered if that's because I've never explored the possibility that I could be. Was I really born sexually uninterested in men? Or had I internalized a social norm to such a degree that I could no longer choose accurately?

Although Jake has "limited" himself to wonderful sexual and romantic experiences with women, he has "kissed a few men in my life." But these were only pecks while playing spin the bottle. When boys had to kiss each other during the game, he and his friends viewed it "as a burden, a penalty . . . A man was supposed to be rigid, strong and masculine and follow the rules of a heteronormative life. So that's what I did." There were no out gays in Jake's high school, and a guy could expect mocking and rebuke if he stepped outside mainstream culture. If there was any sexual experimentation, it had to be with women and not men. Jake wonders, "Is it too late to explore my sexuality?"

Perhaps Jake is slightly late in questioning the totality of his sexuality, but he is not completely out of step with the young men in this book who share their adolescent and young-adult same-sex explorations and yearnings. Many concluded, as Jake did, that their primary sexual and romantic desires remain with women.

Although we don't know enough about Jake to guess his sexuality, are Ezra, Freddie, and Jack mostly straight? Perhaps. Like Josh, each has advocated broad acceptance of various sexualities and romantic orientations. I suspect there are many people in the public eye who are mostly straight; perhaps there are hundreds or thousands. We know that there are many young men in all walks of life who do publicly identify as mostly straight. One of these young men is Dillon.

dillon

*I'm into the Beats like Ginsburg, Burrows, Kerouac, and
they can explain partnerships with males very well, and it is true
in a way. I've had those close companionships.* (DILLON, AGE 20)

DILLON VOLUNTEERED for my Friends and Lovers research
project (for more information, see Appendix A) when he was a
college junior, age 20. Just over a year later, now 22, Dillon completed a scheduled follow-up survey and then asked if he could
come in for an interview to update me on his life. At the same
time, he also participated in a lab study to assess his pupil dilation (which reveals sexual arousal) to erotic images of female and
male porn stars. A year later, at age 23, Dillon said he'd like to
talk with me after visiting a local friend. We met at his favorite
campus hangout. Nearly five years later, when he was 27, Dillon
was again in town, and we met for over an hour to catch up on
his life. As I was finishing my final edits for this book I talked
with him again—he is now 28—by phone, and he responded to
several questions I posed by email. These five interviews, two
surveys, one email, and one lab study are the basis for Dillon's
life history in this book.

Dillon would agree with Josh about everything he said in his media interviews. Dillon identifies as mostly straight, though not in the same way as Josh does. Dillon would more likely want to kiss and cuddle with a guy than to have sex with him. However, if the right guy came along, well, as Dillon sheepishly told me, mirroring Josh, "You just never know . . ."

THE INTERVIEW

Dillon was so eager to tell his story that he stayed beyond the ninety minutes he had reserved on his BlackBerry, and then he asked if he could come back for the chance to tell me more. We scheduled his return, and he shook my hand four times in the process of leaving (twice more after the second interview). Besides being remarkably polite, Dillon was reflective, with a killer smile and an at-ease quality devoid of anxiety or nervousness—somewhat unusual for the young men who volunteered for these interviews. Nothing felt rehearsed for Dillon. It was as if each topic brought forth another triumph, as if he was discovering his life as he considered each question. Dillon wanted this process, these interviews, to help him figure himself out.

Dillon came to the interview with a faux-hawk haircut that was shorter than David Beckham's and the compulsory untied shoes, skinny jeans, and a Jackson Pollock jersey. He certainly wasn't what I expected when he wrote on his pre-interview questionnaire "varsity hockey athlete." Though there was a jockish quality to his mannerisms and physique, there was also a gentleness about him that became quite engaging during the interview. Was he just being exceptionally cool, a metrosexual clone, or something else? It is easy to assume that a hockey player, especially a goalie, is straight, right? Hockey is a rough, bashing, man-to-man contact sport where concussions aren't uncommon. Dillon was a team-sport athlete, a jock, and a guy who said without apology and with conviction that his entire developmental history is traditionally heterosexual. We would soon revisit that assumption.

CHILDHOOD

Dillon grew up in a small, rural Ohio town, the older of two boys in a middle-class family. His father left the family when

Dillon was 15. Until fourth grade, Dillon went to a Montessori school, but he was profoundly unhappy and had few friends. "I'd get so sick I would throw up, probably because I hated leaving home. I had no playmates." Needing more structure, a private all-boys Catholic school was his parents' answer. They were right: Dillon flourished in the new environment, quickly meeting new friends.

Dillon's first distinct sexual memory was hearing from second-grade boys about "playing with their genitalia." That wasn't the word they used, but Dillon knew what they meant, and he soon followed suit. Dillon discovered how wonderful it felt. He didn't exactly know what he was supposed to do, but it just felt fantastic. Thereafter, he humped things, "playing with myself . . . No idea what it was, just felt good. Humping things at school and at home, on desks, poles." Dillon offered another sexual memory: a second-grade girl sitting with him in the back of the bus as they showed each other their "private parts." It was mostly looking, but there was some touching, if only briefly. For Dillon, it was exciting—not monumentally so, but certainly memorable.

Childhood girl crushes soon followed, with the usual success rate for boys of his age. Dillon's first crush was in third grade for a fifth grader, Patty, who at first responded in a positive manner and then became upset, saying, "I'm not your girlfriend!" Patty was older, taller, and growing into her physique: "Brown hair and I liked the connection we had. Pretty girl!" Dillon was uncertain, though, about the feelings he was having and why he was attracted to her.

In the Montessori school he had been neither an outcast nor the most popular. Dillon joined in with his new friends at the Catholic school, who had already connected through team sports. He soon established a core group of buddies, including Bob, a guy today who remains Dillon's best friend. The strong bond among the guys still exists: they would sleep together in the same bed and futon, but they would rarely "talk about it" because some people would think such behavior was "unthinkable." With team sports Dillon had access to status and male bonding. His life improved immeasurably through hockey, baseball, soccer, football, and lacrosse—all sports, all the time. This is the "Dillon" that Dillon loves today.

ADOLESCENCE

Adolescence was a good time for Dillon, especially socially. Dillon came out of his shell, branched out, and gathered new friends. He had Bob, a core group of friends, male comradery, and the intimacy he had longed for. Playing video games, skateboarding, and sitting together during lunch, his friends were "real down to earth" with the same humor and attitudes about girls. This contrasted with other guys in school who "were jerks and had their own parties."

Because he was athletic and worked out on a regular basis, Dillon rated himself as masculine, though he tried to stay "cultured in the arts." By junior year, all barriers to popularity were broken when Dillon began his own jazz band, starred in two varsity sports, joined the ski club, edited the school's literary magazine, and partied and roamed around the neighborhood with friends looking for "female companionship." Dillon wouldn't change a thing about his "awesome" high school years. The one negative, however, was failing to find the intimacy he longed for with girls.

In terms of physical development, Dillon remembered that in fifth grade the Catholic boys were shown a video on how their bodies would change, but the priest said nothing about orgasms or what Dillon was hearing from friends about "the penis going into the vagina." A year later when Dillon was in sixth grade his parents covered the same ground with their version of the sex talk, which was "uncomfortable. I told them that I knew this already." At the time, none of it made much sense to Dillon.

Dillon recalled waking up in seventh grade with "morning wood" and lots of vivid sex dreams. "Sometimes I'd tell my best friend [Bob] as we'd compare similar situations, and share dreams." Dillon couldn't recall any wet dreams, but he definitely noticed an increased degree of being attracted to girls and their physique—not, he self-consciously clarified, "to the point of being a sex addict."

With puberty came wet masturbations with images of "how you could do more things with girls . . . I always kept to myself about masturbation and realized that it was just a natural way of being." Internet porn waited until eighth grade—and, of course, for the adolescent athlete there was the *Sports Illustrated* swimsuit issue. All assisted Dillon's newly energized sexual career. All he needed were the right opportunities and the right girls to make it happen. He never considered boys were in the mix.

DATING AND SEX

The following summer, Dillon's ultimate fantasy was realized while playing Truth or Dare at a friend's birthday party. He was flirting with a cute girl—he can't remember her name, but they were paired, and the dare was taken. Dillon received a hand job from the girl. "It was almost too much but felt awesome. She dared me to finger her, but I didn't, though she wanted me to. I felt embarrassed because [I] didn't know what to do."

In high school, Dillon had many opportunities for vaginal intercourse, but he seized none of them, with no regrets because he feared the girl would know he was a virgin. Besides, Dillon wanted his first time to be within a meaningful relationship. Dating a virgin girl for eight months during his freshman year almost worked out. "We talked about it and decided no . . . We got to the point of attempting to have sex. Both of us were virgins, and she knew my true personality and character and me her."

Then sophomore year he dated a girl for a month off and on. "I was really attached to her, but she was a whore and had slept with 50–60 guys. We dated and she offered sex, and I told her I was a virgin and that was a turnoff to her. I didn't say 'no,' but she just blew it off. I really liked her but wondered where it'd go." Dillon began to fear he might never have sex.

Thus, Dillon was a virgin freshman year of college, but he committed himself to ending this plague. "I thought I was the only one, but I discovered other guys were also virgins. I went to third base several times but never happened. Having sex opened up my mind and finally my desires and sex coming together. Was it just going to be good interactions or just a hookup?" Now that he's had sex twice, "I want more."

Dillon's first time was with a friend of a friend. Five minutes into a movie in her dorm room she initiated the making out. They barely finished before the fire alarm went off.

> This girl was more jumpy and aggressive and had lots of experience. I wanted it to be a meaningful relationship before I did it, but this was a random hookup that lasted one night. She thought I had had sex. She was a freshman and had done it four times. She initiated it. I thought this would be a fast hookup. I loved it and had no regrets. I'm glad it happened. Would like to have meaningful sex sometime . . . We began making out, and we went from there. I almost couldn't see it coming. I just said, "I'm going for it." She had the condom. We had just finished when the fire alarm went off. I had an orgasm, and she said that she did. Sex was great but the relationship wasn't great because [it was] all based on sex. I did need that.

In terms of his future, Dillon labeled his current phase as one of "fucking girls," but then he'd like to become attached.

> But I'm still shopping around. What I want is fucking and short relationships. I've seen lots of girls so far with short flings. I'm also searching for mini-romantic relationships and wait[ing] for the long-term one. With the girls, it is a mixed bag. They want small relationships, not a fling or sex but not to be too intimate right now.
>
> Never had a sweetheart in high school. In the church group, I couldn't do that because the focus was on marriage. I tried to meet as many girls as possible, to experiment. In high school the MO is sex. Girls would take off their top and that was far as they wanted to go. I wondered what I missed in high school.
>
> I've had theory and thoughts about how it has to be a certain someone out there but has to be at the right time. Yes, it is out there, and I guess I'm looking. I'm preoccupied with academics, hockey, and girls—in that order. True love will just happen.

Dillon's relationships with girls haven't worked out. One was only about sex ("the relationship sucked"), and the other, lasting just under a year, ultimately fell apart. "We talked about our future, and we might cross paths again. I saw her over the summer and we made out but not have sex." Until then, Dillon is into "screwing girls" while looking for the *right one*.

SEXUAL AND ROMANTIC STATUS

At this point in the interview I assumed I was talking with a totally straight guy, though one who countered several stereotypes I had about male athletes on an elite hockey team. In retrospect, there were clues—including Dillon's remarkable commitment to male/male intimacy and the ribbing he received in high school and college that he must be gay because of his attention to fashion, especially in styling his hair. He worked part-time one summer as a waiter and a coworker asked Dillon if he was gay. "He was a bit squirrelly, older. He said he was open, and he thought I was gay because of my interactions." This self-reflection was the first indication Dillon might not see himself as exclusively into women. Though Dillon repeatedly accentuated he *definitely* likes women, I was both surprised and intrigued by this admission, as he himself appeared to be.

As I attempted to better understand Dillon's stance, a definitive clarification never came, reflecting Dillon's own ambiguity. Had he ever had genital contact with a guy? "No."

R: Why not?

Don't know. Never opposed to gay interactions. I've joked about it with my friends. I got close once but never made out, though we were physical. One could do homosexual things but not be homosexual.

R: Are you straight?

Don't know. Never had the question before. I've got the testosterone and the masculinity and the attraction to girls. Being gay has crossed my mind, but I wouldn't say that I am. I've had gay friends and an older gay neighbor. People have asked me because I'm a metrosexual in dress and hair, especially this past year.

I have attractions to guys, but it's not sexual. It's my dress, appearance, personality. I've not been intimate, and gay culture is very intimate. A small group of us went to gay bars at home, and it was interesting, a different culture. Mom has gay friends and neighbors, and she is accepting of it, and the culture is very interesting. I'm into the Beats like Ginsburg, Burrows, Kerouac, and they can explain partnerships with males very well, and it is true in a way. I've had those close companionships.

R: How do you see your sexual and romantic development during these college years?

Still definitely attracted to women. I've been curious about my attraction to guys. I wouldn't say I was bi or that I wanted sex with guys—but maybe a relationship guy / guy I'm leaning toward. Not sexual intercourse with a guy [though] I know it would be interesting. I'd try it because [I'd] curious in the future.

A guy on my floor thought I was gay. I am what I am, and that is interesting. Like on the Kinsey scale where 10 was very masculine and 1 very feminine and 5 is bisexual, I'm a 7 or 8. I've thought about the Beats and that I'd like to be like them perhaps.

R: In your ideal future, what would you like to be?

Definitely women still my top priority, and I'd like to have more sex with girls. Maybe I'd like to meet a guy a little more similar to me. A partnership with my feeling homosexual, not acting on it sexually or physically. I know here and there I'd like to be affectionate but not having sex.

R: Do you express affection to other guys?

Not difficult for me to express by hugging and even cuddling with a guy, especially if we are on the same wavelength. I'm not weirded out with little touches. I don't care if people say I'm gay because I hug my best friend. No hesitancy, if appropriate, if I tell a guy that he is sexy and looks good. I've even done it the past week. I act that way more with guys I really know and will do this with my gay friend.

R: How did you get to be attracted to guys?

It depends on how you are raised. I heard that something is different if growing up attracted to guys. Maybe genetics has some role. More needs to be done . . . I've never heard of bisexual guys liking sex with girls, and I'm definitely into liking sex with girls! I'm straight because of the way I was raised, in sports. I'm leaning bisexual, my gay side. Mom raised me to play the piano and guitar, do arts, and that may be a factor . . .

Don't understand females because things get so complicated. With guys you fight and make up in a day, but girls take longer.

Throughout the interview it was difficult to find any evidence that Dillon is homophobic, and any notion that he might be was met with reasoned and passionate denial.

[It's] just wrong to go against someone because of their sexual orientation. I don't go against because I'm afraid they'd be turned on to me. [I was] raised knowing gay people . . . Doesn't seem weird to me to see guys kissing, and my parents are accepting of them. My core group of friends influenced me not to be homophobic and comfortable with each other . . .

I have dated two bisexual females which was okay with me. They both go more for guys but will play with girls. They can do this more than guys can. I have no interest in girl-on-girl action. If in serious relationship I wonder what if she found a girl she wanted to be with, best of both worlds. Girls like that. They don't like headstrong masculine testosterone males.

MUSINGS

Based on his heterosexual desires, sex with women, romantic relationships with women, and a masculine gender role, it would be easy to label Dillon as straight. Except what should we make of his frequent references to same-sex romantic desires and his willingness, at least his curiosity, to try out sex with guys? Aren't straight guys supposed to give up their passionate child and adolescent boyhood friendships once they enter the adult world of heterosexuality? And, unlike straight guys, Dillon doesn't deny a "gay side" to himself.

Supporting the mostly straight option, Dillon is sexually progressive in his attitudes, admittedly an outlier among his hockey teammates. Dillon has never known a gay hockey player, and there are lots of gay jokes and references in the shower room about the size and shape of each other's penis. For Dillon, guys are physically and sexually attractive, but though he has kissed a guy he's gone no further. If circumstances were ever right, however, it might happen. But what most distinguished Dillon as a mostly straight traveler was his longing for emotionally intimate relationships with guys.

Throughout his life Dillon has had boy chums, crushes, and infatuations with teammates, band members, and best friends. Within the sports context Dillon revels in touching and being touched, experiencing pats to the butt, arms around the shoulder, and fist and crotch bumps. While watching movies and eating popcorn, Dillon has cuddled with guy friends, especially if they are on the same wavelength. Dillon could meet a guy and together develop a partnership. They wouldn't necessarily act on it sexually, but they'd be physically affectionate and trust each other. Dillon isn't naïve, and he knows their relationship would be difficult for others to understand. It'd be labeled gay because of the time he and his partner would spend together, the secrets they'd share, and the knowing glances, nods, and code words they'd exchange. This is the "homosexual thing" that most interests Dillon.

Even in today's progressive youth culture, it is remarkable that Dillon is so utterly unbothered if others think he's gay. It's an unproblematic curiosity for Dillon. Seeing guys kiss doesn't weird him out. It does his friends. He doesn't care if gays are turned on by him. It does his friends. Might these differences mean something? Dillon isn't sure. Although he has gay friends, goes to gay bars, and reads gay writers, other straight young men of his generation do as well. And they also believe it is simply wrong to discriminate against someone because of his sexual orientation. In this they dramatically depart from previous generations.

Whether Dillon's guy attractions are rooted in an admiration of masculine beauty, his father leaving, or a sexually discrete if coy turn-on is never completely clear to me. Dillon deftly turned aside such questions, but glowed when he announced "Why, just this past week I told a guy he was looking good, looking sexy." Not wanting to be so easily thwarted, I asked, "You mean in a sexual kind of way?" And, here, Dillon gave another non-answer:

"If the guy is attractive enough . . . You just never know." Maybe this answer is the essence of mostly straightness—you just never know. By his own admission, Dillon resides in the sexual never-lands, a place between heterosexuality and bisexuality.

Dillon is part of a growing trend of young men secure in their heterosexuality and yet aware of their potential for experiencing far more. We'll return to Dillon throughout the book, especially toward the end when he talks more about his life after college.

To remind us as we move forward: Mostly straight men are heterosexual, with a slight dose of same-sex sexuality that can be either sexual, romantic, or both. How is this possible? Through their life stories, the mostly straight young men will tell us. Far more than we realize, young men wait to be released from heterosexual straightjackets. Dillon might just show us the way.

sexual and romantic spectrums

Well, people really like to think of the [sexual] world
as in black and white, and really it's all grey. (RYAN, AGE 23)

WHEN I ASKED DILLON IF HE'S STRAIGHT, he couldn't give
me an unequivocal, "Yes." Rather, the standard categories don't
fit him; he's neither straight nor gay. "I've got the testosterone
and the masculinity and the attraction to girls. Being gay has
crossed my mind, but I wouldn't say that I am." And bisexual
didn't fit either. Dillon is lost in the world of categories and ab-
solutes. Dillon is on the spectrum, the Kinsey continuum.

In the 1940s, sex researcher Alfred Kinsey defied the pervasive orthodoxy of a dichotomous, either-or perspective toward
sexual orientation. His counterproposition was a 7-point *con-*
tinuum, ranging from exclusively heterosexual (Kinsey 0) to
exclusively homosexual (Kinsey 6). In this scheme, mostly heterosexuals are Kinsey 1s and primarily heterosexuals, I would
suppose, are Kinsey 0.5s. Kinsey did not provide sexual identity
names—straight, bisexual, gay—to these numbers because he
was assessing sexual orientation, which we now understand to be
the relative degree of sexual attraction an individual has for men,

for women, or for both. The key for a continuum perspective is to append the words "to varying degrees" to all components of sexuality, including sexual attraction, desire, arousal, and behavior. Sexual identity, whether consistent or not with sexual orientation, is the name or label an individual applies to that sexuality.

Despite Kinsey's continuum framework, we refer to sexual orientation and sexual identity in categorical terms: one is either straight, bisexual, gay, or lesbian. Whether sexuality should be conceptualized as a continuum as Kinsey imagined it, with degrees of attractions to women and men, or as three discrete categories as sex scholars currently envision it remains an unresolved controversy.

These two approaches have been branded *lumping,* those who reduce sexuality to its bare minimum, and *splitting,* those who emphasize overlapping qualities among the lumpers' categories. Lumpers combine Kinsey 0s and 1s and define them as straight. The Kinsey 5s and 6s become gay/lesbian. All extraneous (nonexclusive) orientations (Kinsey 2s, 3s, and 4s) are labeled bisexual. Although splitters don't have names for all possibilities along the continuum, they reject any approach that labels all nonexclusives as "bisexual" because it lumps together some very odd bedfellows. For example, imagine that a guy who has twenty female and two male sex partners is in the same bisexual category as another guy who has two female and twenty male sex partners.

Although lumpers combine Kinsey 0s and 1s and label them as straight individuals, I side with the splitters. For me, Kinsey 1s are in between Kinsey 0s (exclusive heterosexuals) and Kinsey 2s (bisexual-leaning heterosexuals), and I refer to them as mostly heterosexuals. In a sense, mostly heterosexuality (the sexual orientation term) is a form of bisexuality, but a mostly straight (the sexual identity term) individual resides on the extreme left side of bisexuality, just inches from heterosexuality.

Both lumpers and splitters usually agree that the vast majority of young men congregate at the extreme ends of the continuum—they're either straight or gay. I'll readily concede that most young men are straight; some would say 90 to 95 percent, but I would guess that the percentage is closer to 80 if one removed mostly straight guys from the equation. Gay young men constitute around 5 percent of the population. The point of greatest contention is the number of young men who place themselves at neither end of the continuum. Although the precise number of these in-betweens is unknown, mostly straight is a substantial class, far greater than we might assume. Perhaps over 10 percent of the U.S. male population is mostly straight. That's millions of guys.

romantic orientation

[It's] not difficult for me to express by hugging and even
cuddling with a guy, especially if we are on the
same wavelength. (DILLON, AGE 20)

TO UNDERSTAND SEXUALITY, we need to make a distinction between the sexual and romantic aspects of our lives. That is sometimes difficult to do. Although we might desire a *sexual union* with another, we might not desire a *romantic union* with that person. The sexual and the romantic are usually strongly associated with each other, but they're not identical. For most young men, the gender they fall in love is the gender they have sex with. This is where mostly straights complicate the picture. Nearly all have a slight degree of discrepancy between their sexual and romantic lives. For example, Dillon fervently wants sex with women, but he also craves romance with a guy.

A relatively new field, relationship science, can help us understand two primary aspects of romantic orientation. *Passionate love* is having an intense craving for uniting with another. When it is reciprocated, a young man feels fulfilled and ecstatic. When it is unrequited, however, he experiences separation anxiety, emptiness, and despair. In common jargon, passionate love is a crush, infatuation, puppy love, limerence, and being in love. Young children, both boys and girls beginning as young as 3 years, are as likely as early adolescents to experience passionate love.

The second aspect of romantic orientation is *companionate love,* a cluster of feelings that includes romantic intimacy, attachment, and commitment. When a young man experiences companionate love, he desires close, emotional proximity with the object of his desires. In the presence of this person, he feels calmness, social comfort, and security. If this closeness is threatened, separation anxiety again surfaces. Although perhaps first experienced as an adolescent, *true love* more commonly is a feature of late adolescence and young adulthood.

An individual can have one or both types of love, and one can evolve into the other. Both are universal, biological phenomena rooted in our species' physiology to promote bonding with other people and mating (procreation) success. Supporting this view, passionate love and companionate love have been documented across historical time and a considerable number of cultural groups. From an evolutionary perspective, if you want to improve your chances of passing along your genes to future generations, it might be advantageous to form a bond with the person you'd like to mate with. This union will likely increase production success through enhanced care for the merchandise—children.

Perhaps ironically, during our prehistory bonding with same-sex others also improved fitness. It allowed women to mutually care for and protect their children and to develop agriculture while men were out gathering protein. In turn, becoming attached with other men enhanced men's hunting skills and success through cooperation and joint efforts. Indeed, one could argue that the state of mostly heterosexuality served an evolutionary purpose: such individuals had the heterosexuality to motivate mating and the homosexuality to create bonds with same-sex others. Having other men for sexual pleasure and romantic security while the sexes were separated could have promoted the survival of our species.

Although we should have known that the romantic overlapped with the sexual without necessarily being identical parts of who we are, it took a group of fifty adolescents of varied sexualities to remind us. In focus groups, they were asked to define sexual orientation. Across multiple gender and sexual expressions and identities, they reached a consensus in two parts. They defined sexual orientation as sexual attraction: an intense, physiological reaction to one's preferred sex. It's what turns your head in the school lunchroom or gym. You feel yourself on edge, energized when an attractive member of your preferred sex is in the room. But that's not all. Sexual orientation is also about romantic attraction, which usually commences with a crush that the object of your affection might or might not know about or want, and moves to being or desiring to be in love with and form a long-term commitment with someone of your preferred sex.

For many youths, love and sex are difficult to differentiate. Sometimes they're linked, as in, "I can only (or, want to) have sex with a woman if I'm in love with her." Other times the two correspond, almost: "I only fall in love and have sex with women, but wouldn't mind going down on a guy." And sometimes the two are not at all connected, as in having hookup sex with one sex and crushes on the other. That said, for most youths the sync between sexual and romantic intimacy is consistent, if not for the same person then for the same gender.

To help the young men I interviewed sort through these possibilities, I asked each about his sexual and romantic orientations during childhood, middle school, high school, and young adulthood. Then we explored what each of them meant and how they have been expressed.

> Please write down the percentage of your sexual attraction, sexual fantasy, sexual behavior, infatuation, and romantic relationship is to females and what percentage is to males. The total for each domain should be 100 percent.

In a perfect world of simplicity, all five domains would be the same—100 percent toward females (straight) or males (gay). And they probably are for most young men, but not all. Included in the "not all" category are mostly straight young men.

sexual and romantic fluidity

I'm not completely heterosexual. I like to think of myself as fluid.
I have man crushes when a male is so cool . . . I like the idea of male fluidity.
(MOSTLY STRAIGHT YOUTH, AGE 21)

IN RECENT YEARS, we've heard a lot about *sexual fluidity*. A range of publications—from *Glamour* and the *Wall Street Journal* to *Slate* online—have explained, sensationalized, and even touted the merits of sexual fluidity, frequently with little clarity about what it is. What is indisputable is that when they say "fluidity" they mean "women." Rarely are men described as fluid in their sexual or romantic desires.

Both lumpers and splitters agree that female sexuality is substantially more flexible, fluid, and shaped by sociocultural factors such as women's studies classes and female friendships. Male sexuality, by contrast, is considered more rigid, stable, and shaped by biological factors such as genetics and prenatal hormones. Men are supposedly sexually categorical, either straight or gay.

I disagree, and so do the men in this book. My view diverges in two respects:

1. Young men can be sexually fluid in the same way and at the same rate (which is unknown, for either sex) as young women.
2. Fluidity should not be restricted to sexual domains but should also include romantic aspects. A young man may be sexually or romantically fluid, or both.

To be clear regarding definitions, according to experts who study such matters, sexual fluidity has three meanings:

1. An increased capacity for erotic responses to one's nonpreferred sex (such as to males for straight men).
2. Erotic responses depend on the context.
3. Changes during one's lifetime in what is erotic.

Mostly straight youth are sexually or romantically fluid in that, consistent with the first meaning, they have the capacity for erotic and romantic responses to other males, their nonpreferred sex. They either defined themselves as mostly straight or said that less than 100 percent of their sexual and romantic attractions are to women.

The second definition also applies to the life narratives you will soon read. Although I did not specifically ask each young man about inconsistencies in his erotic and romantic arousal, these variations will be evident as each young man narrates his developmental history. For example, his sexual preference might change if it is partnered sex (only with females) versus group sex (now he'll play with males). He might have sexual fantasies or romantic crushes with feminine but not masculine men—or the opposite. And to complicate matters, most of these men are fluid in their sexual or romantic life, but not in both.

The third definition, variability over time, was assessed for a subset of the youths but only for about eighteen months. I also asked each young man to recall his sexual and romantic development during early, middle, and late adolescence. As we'll see later, nearly all attested to fulfilling this condition of fluidity. They have swapped portions of their sexuality and romantic inclinations, if not in their sexual identity then certainly in the percentage of sexual and romantic attractions devoted to each sex. These changes can also be witnessed in the life narratives when the young men relate how their romantic and sexual feelings evolved, especially from adolescence to young adulthood.

Few of these fluctuations were conscious choices the guys made; rather, they were the result of a growing reflection on their true self. Most felt their fluidity was a natural feature of their self-development. Certainly they could choose whether to tolerate the attractions and whether to engage in sexual or romantic behavior that reflected their fluidity. And, of course, some were more motivated to make these changes than others. Whether they were born with the capacity to be fluid or weren't didn't especially concern them. My answer to what causes fluidity, the relative degrees of biology and social/cultural context, is simply, "We don't know." And the young men didn't care.

Will, a youth we'll soon meet, believes we should simply acknowledge the existence of fluidity. On his eighteen-month follow-up questionnaire, Will wrote, "I think there should be much more fluidity in how we talk about sexual categories. I think people should develop a keener historical sense of how these categories came to be as they are."

it is who i am

A guy on my floor thought I was gay.
I am what I am, and that is interesting. (DILLON, AGE 20)

IF YOU DOUBT THAT A BOY OR YOUNG MAN can be mostly straight, listen carefully to their life histories. They tell us a mostly straight identity is subjectively meaningful to them and authentically reflects their romantic and sexual desires. Their stories are difficult to discount. They're not trying to be someone else, to fake us out, or to confuse us. It is who they are.

The significance of mostly heterosexuality for youths' lives has become progressively more obvious and widespread during the past decade. I lead youth workshops on sexuality, and I've been impressed with the resolute and unwavering way the teen participants snub traditional sexual labels. In these workshops, I have an exercise in which they write on a notecard how they describe or identify their sexuality to themselves. The responses are inspired, blunt, bizarre, inventive, and, on many occasions, funny. One wrote, "I like what I like regardless of what's down their pants. If someone's attractive, they're attractive. The end. No identity." In a similar brusque yet candid manner, a 16-year-old boy wrote, "I don't desire to identify my sexuality. I just am me. Get over it."

When they "followed directions," the teens responded with descriptions about their sexuality that might appear unrecognizable to many of us but are, in many circumstances, quite thoughtful. Here are two 16-year-old boys at the gay end of the sexual/romantic continuum:

- "Faggot!! The best! Sexy, hot, beautiful, intimate."
- "I also connect with women, emotionally much more easily than I do men. This presents a significant obstacle in terms of partners. My life would be a lot different in terms of sex/relationships if I were at all aroused by women, but I'm not (to my considerable chagrin, I might add). You might say I live by the (very true!) adage, 'a good man is hard to find.'"

Most of the workshop boys were trying to figure it out and wanted to communicate their struggles. Certainly they didn't want to be reduced to a sexual category because they didn't capture the complexity of what they were going through. But it wasn't just boys primarily attracted to the same sex who were trying to find their way through adult-oriented sexual and romantic categories. Some straight-identified boys, though privileged to have the sexuality that predominates in America, were open to reconsideration—they're not "blind" to good-looking guys but are "open-minded" and "love who I love."

- "I am straight to the present. I can be attracted to girls, and I have had relationships with only girls but maybe I haven't met the right guy yet. Right now, I am straight, but open to possibilities, depending on what happens next."
- "Straight, but not narrow. I have had relationships with only straight identifying females. I have thought (extensively) about my sexuality, and thus far I am attracted, emotionally and sexually, to females."

What are they telling us? Are they on their way to becoming "something else"? Are they "bisexuals in disguise" or "progressive heterosexuals"? These are difficult questions to answer because we traditionally identify these youth as bisexuals, questioning, or "others," or we delete them altogether because we don't know what to do with them. Either we disbelieve them or, equally bad, dismiss their experienced sexuality. Perhaps we'll never understand, but we owe it to them to at least try to make sense of their past and present sexual and romantic reflections. We should listen.

Granted, when a youth identifies as something "in between" that doesn't have widespread recognition or acceptance, it can make his life more challenging. He might thus experience an ongoing process of sexual and romantic exploration, which likely distinguishes him from many of his straight peers.

I now turn to youths who most threaten the concept of mostly straightness—young men who say they're straight but acknowledge an extremely slight degree of same-sex sexuality. This will lead us to consider mostly straight young men who identify as such not because of their sexuality but because of their progressive politics.

straight, but not totally straight

I'm not ashamed that I'm not gay.
(PRIMARILY STRAIGHT YOUTH, AGE 22)

IN EVERY CENTURY AND CULTURE for which we have sufficient information, some straight-identified men have sexual
contact or an infatuation with another guy. It's usually a small
number, less than 5 percent of straight guys; nevertheless, this
represents millions of young men. For example, in a U.S. national
study released in 2016, 2.8 percent of self-identified heterosexual
men, ages 18 to 44, reported that they had engaged in same-sex
behavior. Of course, this is likely an underestimate. Other cases
were likely missed because a straight man decided whatever he
had done with another man didn't count as sex (such as receiving a blow job) or he was not going to report the sexual encounter because he didn't trust the confidentiality of the survey.

Another striking finding, from a recent study of over 8,000
youth between the ages of 15 and 24, is that over 20 percent reported having some degree of same-sex attraction, behavior, or
identity, yet they identified as straight—even if they currently had

a male sex partner. It is also noteworthy that of those who reported having any sexual attraction to males, nearly half said they were attracted "mostly to females."

If you were to take all teenage boys and young adult men who have ever had sex (usually defined as oral or anal sex) with another male, the majority, around 60 percent, currently identifiy as straight. For example, in a recent national study of Australians, nearly two-thirds of men who have had sex with both women and men currently identify not as bisexual or gay, as you might expect, but as straight.

What's going on? The title of one article says it all: "Straight Men Are a Lot More Bisexual Than You Might Think." Without doubt this is true for some men—closeted gay or bisexual men pretending to be straight but wanting gay sex. Or on gay or bisexual apps and websites men might feign straightness to be perceived as more attractive to potential male sex partners (or to fulfill their own fantasy). Are there other possibilities?

Clearly young men have the capacity to maintain a straight identity in the face of having sex with guys. Why would a straight guy have gay sex? I'm not sure—because we seldom ask him. The usual suspects, at least ones I've heard from straight guys I've interviewed, include:

- I was only experimenting or was curious.
- I was drunk or high and don't remember what happened.
- It was a favor to a friend because he was depressed or was attracted to me.
- It was a dare (Truth-or-Dare game) or a fraternity or athletic ritual.
- I needed the money.
- I was in prison, a boarding school, or the military where girls/women weren't available.
- Hey, any orgasm is an orgasm, especially if you keep your eyes shut.

Without ruling out or casting judgment about these reasons, I offer another possibility: perhaps it is an authentic expression of his sexuality. And for such a young man we have a unique place for him on the sexual continuum—inbetween exclusively straight and mostly straight. In the future, he may conceivably identify as mostly straight, or he may want to preserve the ambiguity, identifying truthfully as straight while maintaining a small degree of same-sex attraction, behavior, or both.

In terms of romantic orientation, it's also possible that he has no sexual attraction to men or has never had sex with men but does have guy crushes and, perhaps, has been in love with a guy. He might argue that these are normal guy things and thus not indicative of anything other than what he is:

- It's a boy crush. He's my best buddy.
- Lots of people cuddle with a warm body while watching a movie.
- We were kissing and showing affection to entice the girls, to turn them on.
- I'm a metrosexual kind of guy.
- It's just a bromance. Lots of guys have them with each other.

Such an individual might interpret his small degree of same-sex sexuality as within the bounds of heterosexuality. His sexual or romantic tendencies toward other men are too sparse to qualify as anything other than heterosexual and are not so prevalent to qualify him as mostly straight—which might seem too bisexual for him. Or he doesn't interpret his same-sex desires as a general attribute of his sexuality but instead sees them as specific to a very small number of particular guys (such as a best friend), or to a type of guy (such as muscular men), or in select situations (such as experimenting with what receiving oral sex from an expert feels like). Or, as one young man explained, to help him teach his girlfriend techniques for giving good head.

Perhaps if it weren't for the still-present social stigma against acknowledging any same-sex sexuality, he might label such feelings or experiences as mostly straight. By identifying as straight, any sexual or romantic deviations from total straightness are deemed inconsequential for his self-identity or for his standing among friends and family. In this respect, he differs from a mostly straight guy.

WHO IS STRAIGHT, BUT NOT TOTALLY STRAIGHT?

Simply, a straight but not totally straight young man identifies as straight (not mostly straight) but has a very small, perhaps 1 to 2 percent, degree of same-sex attraction. One young man came to the interview on crutches due to an athletic injury. He identifies as straight but not exclusively straight, including both sexual and romantic aspects.

> I think there have been times where I have had small, little attraction to guys. Nothing that I wanted to act upon, but just little attractions, I guess. I think whenever I come really close to a guy like as a friend, there will always be a time, not that I look up to them, just like I admire them for having everything together and just probably a little physical part to it too. Just a compilation of all of that. Just a step past admiring how close I am to them.

He acknowledges that he is not absolutely heterosexual in all respects. Of course, it's possible he's in denial about his sexual and romantic attractions in terms of their prevalence, intensity, or frequency, or they may have been more meaningful than he's prepared to grant. However, it is also possible he is being entirely truthful.

Unwittingly, he and other young men like him cast further doubt on absolute sexual categories. Perhaps we could place them on sexual and romantic continuums between exclusively heterosexual (Kinsey 0) and mostly heterosexual (Kinsey 1)—perhaps we'll say they are a Kinsey 0.5 and call them *primarily straight*. They share with the other two the same level of sexual and romantic arousal to women, but they diverge from exclusively straight guys by adding a slight degree of same-sex arousal and from mostly straight guys by subtracting a slight degree of same-sex arousal.

These young men seldom provoke gay slurs, with a few exceptions. Two boys I interviewed were teased for rather sketchy reasons—because one was friendly and thin and the other was artistic and liked to sew.

- "Yeah because I was a really nice guy, friendly, outgoing and in ninth grade I lost a lot of weight and was skinny and tall and that made me gay. Being thin and nice, I guess."
- "In junior high some saw me as gay because I was artistic and less into sports and because I sewed better in home economics than most of the girls. This was because my mother was a fashion designer."

Whether primarily straight is a distinct sexuality is not the main point. The point is that within the world of straightness exists a range of normal attractions and responses, which illustrates that being straight is not a singular experience. My preference is to see the athletically injured young man on crutches as he is and place him on our ever-expanding sexual and romantic continuums.

HOW DID HE GET THAT WAY?

Like sexual fluidity, we don't know how straight guys develop a slight degree of same-sex sexuality. We don't know because we don't recognize their existence; we don't think to ask how they got to be the way they are. However, I'll take a few moments to speculate.

One possibility is that a young man was born straight but with the capacity to expand his sexuality into other realms because of his personality traits, such as curiosity, a sense of adventure, and sensation seeking. Another, perhaps related, possibility is he was influenced by random events occurring in his life, such as opportunities to explore his sexual side (playing doctor with a boy) or having role models that he romantically adored (a star athlete who took him under his wing). That is, a primarily straight young man is a straight young man who, because of his openness to new experiences, progressive values system, exposure to gay friends or feminist theory, or all the above, recognizes that he has a slight degree of same-sex sexuality. That little bit is acceptable, intriguing, fun, and daring, especially in this age of increasing gay acceptance. As we interview more youth, we might learn more.

ATTITUDES TOWARD GAYS

One potential consequence of their slight degree of same-sex sexuality is that primarily straight youths have a greater tolerance in general with nonheterosexual sexualities. Overall as a group they were as progressive in their attitudes toward gays and homosexuality as mostly straight men, both of whom were considerably more liberal in this regard than many straight men—and even some gay men.

Although most of the straight men I interviewed favored gay rights, which is in sync with their generation, far fewer were comfortable with my questions regarding same-sex attractions, crushes, and sexual contacts with guys. I made sure to emphasize that I asked the same questions of all guys regardless of their stated sexual identity. Many responded matter-of-factly along the lines of "Not attracted to guys in that way," "Never found it appealing, I guess," or "Doesn't float my boat." Others, however, weren't so kind, with the facial grimace to match:

- "It is revolting to me. If [I] see two males make out, then it turns my stomach."
- "Disgusting. Whole idea grosses me out, and I go back to religion on this."
- "Gross! Way I was raised has a lot to do with it. It's not right and personally it goes against nature."
- "I find it disgusting. I'm still kind of homophobic like maybe jokingly I'll say, like 'that's so gaynice' [does femme impersonation with limp wrists and voice]."

By contrast were the typical responses from the primarily straight young men, who saw advantages to being gay:

- "Gay males have tons of straight female friends, lots of activities on campus are geared toward them, so it's cool to be gay. If [you are] gay and accept it, then freeing and self-actualizing."
- "I have tons of gay friends, and I find it so unthreatening if a guy says he is attracted to me."

One young man, Demetri, who we'll soon meet, sided with mostly straights rather than exclusively straights. Although Demetri recognizes that his sexuality is more geared toward the straight end of the spectrum, he had an explanation for why straight guys might be repulsed by an ounce of same-sex sexuality.

> R: How do you see yourself as different from a straight guy?

> I am definitely not repulsed by any of that [gay sex]. I don't see why people, I don't want to say it's not as normal as heterosexual sex, but I definitely don't think it's strange. I think everyone should be allowed to do whatever they want to do. It's providing the same physical stimulation. It's just done a little differently.

> The people who are like that [repulsed] will never admit it usually. But you can feel it. I can feel the difference, especially if you are in close vicinity to them. If you close your eyes, you can feel people bending the fields around you. You are very sensitive to that. I think it stems from, I think it's more common in athletes, especially people who idealize like a male archetype that's really basically spectacular or whatever. It definitely happens more in people who are mama's boys, I've noticed.

> In my experience, there's two archetypes. There's one archetype who would never admit it and is like the guy's guy, and you can just feel that in certain situations I know you are hiding something here and I don't know why. And there's other people who probably would admit it in the right situation but because of parents or whatever social norm they are trying to fit into won't. But it seems more obvious.

The possibility that Demetri is running away from his slight degree of same-sex sexuality is highly questionable given his progressive nature. And, after all, he voluntarily disclosed his sexual and romantic interest in guys.

Another possibility has less to do with attitudes than with personality characteristics, those I noted previously, of primarily straight youth and their expanded vision of sexuality. They, like mostly straights, express considerable interest in having casual sex with women, and they are sexually curious and open to new experiences. I sensed little reservation from these young men in exploring their same-sex sexuality, and many had—not necessarily behaviorally (sexually) or emotionally (romantically) but cognitively—by thinking, "What if I had sex with a guy?" and "What would it mean if I did?" Few, however, at this point in their lives were willing to forsake their principal focus—sexual and romantic forays with women. After all, this is the time when women are so plentiful, so gorgeous, and so diverse, and opportunities to pursue erotic encounters with them and to search for the special one are so tempting. This isn't the time to try out gay sex.

I'll illustrate with a young man with a thoughtful answer to my question regarding whether he has had genital contact with another male. "No, but I have been at times wondered about, considered it." He defined himself as "heterosexual but open to the possibility of other stuff, whatever." The pull toward men was not sufficiently strong, though he was quick to add, "At the same time I can appreciate the male body." Might he have sex with a guy in the future? He struggled in explaining his position.

> I'm 100 percent attracted to girls, but maybe a small percent of that would apply to guys, but I don't like the idea of lots of sexual interactions and I only want one. Nothing wrong with having intercourse with guys but don't think I necessarily want to try it out just to see.
>
> My only regret, a relatively minor one, is the fact that, yes, I thought about sex with guys but never think I'll see the other side of things, for better or worse. As things stand right now I'm pretty satisfied with my life. Yet I'm vaguely curious, wondering if curiosity is like a valid enough reason to make a change of that magnitude. Maybe the ideal thing, if I want to have the freedom to see what the other side has to offer and bisexuals have that.

Given the varied life experiences of other primarily straight youth, one might wonder if their sexuality will be stable over time.

STABILITY

Maybe a primarily straight youth is merely a mostly straight guy who is in slight denial and is moving in that direction but has not yet arrived. Perhaps once he totally rejects society's lack of comfortableness with same-sex sexuality he'll allow himself to acknowledge a larger degree of sexual and romantic attractions that mostly straight guys endorse. That is, will he stay the way he is now?

I have very limited information to enlighten us. Of the nine primarily straight guys I interviewed, six identified as straight at Time 1 and became primarily straight youth at Time 2, almost two years later. They recalled a slight bit of same-sex sexuality, usually during early adolescence and extending into high school, especially in their masturbatory fantasies, sexual attractions, or infatuations. Their same-sex sexuality generally diminished over time or remained stable. The other three were previously primarily straight youth and remained so during their college years.

I can't answer with any certainty whether these youths will migrate to mostly heterosexuality, reverse themselves to return to exclusive heterosexuality, or stay put. My tentative answer is that they might well fluctuate among these three but essentially will have the capacity to have a slight degree of same-sex sexuality, elicited or acknowledged through biological (personality traits, sex libido) and/or environmental (exposure to liberal attitudes, environmental opportunities) factors. Regardless, they are fundamentally straight men expecting in their future to be heterosexually married with children, with their same-sex sexuality intact but not acted on sexually or romantically. Perhaps they'll have an occasional sexual fling with a guy or an intense male friendship that feels like a crush. We just don't know—yet.

DEVELOPMENTAL TRAJECTORIES

What most strikes me about primarily straight young men is their diversity in developmental trajectories. They diverged among themselves—not all in the same way, at the same time, or to the same degree. Some were aware of their sexual and romantic development, but others were rather clueless, perhaps because no one had ever asked them. When did your same-sex sexuality begin? How did it progress to where it is today? What does it mean? These three youths had remote clues:

- "Never made out, never a crush, but what I felt for Alex [best friend] could be really understood by someone like it was a romantic relationship."
- "If I see a good-looking male, is that sexual attraction? What if two guys and a girl are in the same fantasy? Does that count?"
- "I've thought about what it would be like to be a girl, gay, or bisexual. Fantasized about it."

Nearly all clarified that although they might have a slight degree of sexual or romantic attractions or fantasies involving guys, acting on these was highly unlikely. Fewer than one-fifth has had sexual contact with a male, and that contact has consisted of kissing or making out. If it was genital, then it was during his boyhood. Why had he made out with another male?

- "When almost drunk I kissed a guy in high school but was making fun of his girlfriend in spin the bottle. Then one time I jokingly kissed a friend. Never felt like exploring it that much."
- "Yes, I made out with a guy at a naked party. I was pretty intoxicated, and this gay friend of mine, well we met that night. He helped me go home, and he kissed me. Beard didn't feel good and tasted salty. No meaning for me. I was drunk. Nothing more happened."
- "Kissed a boy in a Truth-or-Dare sort of thing. We're in the hot tub naked with lots of people. No big deal and it didn't mean anything. This was in high school. Honestly, I was a kid, and we talked sexuality a lot so we pined to kiss. We're best friends, so nothing gay about it."
- "As children we'd play gay chicken: How far up do you go on a guy's leg before giving up [touching the genitals]. Experimental and my friend was the best person to do it with. Didn't feel wrong or gay because understood between the two of us what it meant."

Everyone denied any gay intent or interpretation of his actions. He was young, it was fun, and it meant nothing. Or did it? Would a straight youth be willing to participate this far? I suspect some might, but I don't know.

I'm uncertain whether these activities reasonably place a young man at a coherent point along a sexual/romantic spectrum or they constitute a rather loose gathering of diverse activities that mean little except the individual has some small amount of same-sex sexual or romantic interest. To clarify, I asked each in an open-ended format about his sexuality now, a prediction about his future, and ideally how he'd like to be. Each interpreted the question to reflect his personal deliberations about the nature of his sexuality, with considerable ambivalence.

- "No desire to be with a guy but would be open if things came up for me. Wouldn't be any less likely to be happy. So unthreatening to me if a guy says he is attracted to me. Perfectly capable of saying, 'No.' It's no threat to portraying myself as a straight person. My uncle is gay so have had it in my life."
- "People are more sexually open than we allow them to be. I'm hardwired to be straight and never felt a bisexual leaning but a desire to desire it. I'm not ashamed that I'm not gay. It's a part of my socialization."
- "I can appreciate if a male is good-looking. Thought of it in a sexual way in my head but never acted on it. Most of my sexual identity and attractions have been with girls from the beginning, and I feel more fulfilling than when I thought of guys."
- "Once a girl in college asked me if I was gay. I have no discomfort with homosexuality."

A clear theme in these responses is one of incredible comfortableness with same-sex sexuality. It would not be the worst thing to happen to him; in fact, it would be okay if he were gay. True, it didn't turn out that way, but if it had he would be equally happy. He is open to the possibility, but it's not in the cards for now—but it might be. Although several considered pursuing their slight amount of same-sex sexuality, none have done so, at least while sober, during young adulthood.

The question, once again, is whether these guys will pursue same-sex sexuality in the future. The answer is unknown, but what I can say with confidence is that he'll likely be far more likely to do so than his straight brothers. After all, he's blessed with an amazing willingness to be flexible and consider all options. His level of sexual prejudice is quite low, he recognizes the reality of gay life in America, and he's fine with where he is today.

Three young men—Demetri, Ricky, and Chris—give life to what it means to be primarily straight—that is, to identify as straight (Kinsey 0.5), not mostly straight (Kinsey 1.0), and yet have a degree of same-sex sexuality. However, it is a considerably smaller amount of attraction to guys than what the mostly straights report.

demetri

If I were to meet a man who I was attracted to,
I would not be afraid to be attracted to them. (DEMETRI, AGE 19)

THOUGH CLEARLY A UNIQUE INDIVIDUAL, as you will soon discover, Demetri's childhood and adolescence were typically heterosexually oriented, with girl crushes, dates with girls, and early sex with girls. Any indication that he might not be totally straight only emerged during late high school and college. There was something about Demetri that signaled *possibilities,* as gay guys, even in high school, hit on him. Demetri attributed his appeal to his "affectionate warmth." He rated himself as exclusively straight sexually and mostly straight romantically with a classic Josh Hutcherson-like comment: "I am attracted to individuals, and, if I were to meet a man who I was attracted to, I would not be afraid to be attracted to them." That said, Demetri lacks the sexual *burn* for guys, though he has tried "going in" toward them—more on this later.

Tall, lanky, with a slight scruff of a chin beard and longish hair, 19-year-old Demetri thoroughly read the consent form, stopping at points to ask for clarification. He wore black socks, black shoes, shorts from another era that were perhaps purchased at a vintage clothing shop, and a loose-fitting T-shirt. He did not look like your typical college student, an observation that would please him immensely. Demetri was a sophomore chemistry major living in a progressive co-op with his girlfriend of nearly two years, though they were not exclusive with each other.

A waiter at a Southeast Asian café, an environmental activist, and a leader who prefers to operate behind the scenes, Demetri projected his future as one in which he will explore the addictive effects of drugs on brain synapses and pathways, especially the dopamine system. Demetri was adamant that he wouldn't be having children: "Hell, no. I probably won't have children in America. I probably won't have children, period . . . If I wanted to have kids I would need to have them now or in the next year or two." And having those children any time soon is not on Demetri's agenda.

When I completed my set of questions, Demetri looked disappointed, saying I could ask more questions if I wanted to. He also wondered if he could recommend people for the study (and the answer was yes). Demetri reluctantly left. He slowly, deliberately, turned and thanked me profusely.

Typical of straight boys, Demetri's friends were other boys, yet they weren't drawn from team sports but from drama club, band, and cross-country. He felt most relaxed while "chilling with my boys." When I asked Demetri to describe whether he considered himself masculine or feminine, he broke with the typical interview protocol—"Such a funny question." Consistent with the "masculine archetype" that American culture mandates, that men should be "liking women, drinking whiskey, gambling, and shooting guns," Demetri's answer was a resounding, "Yes." To illustrate,

Demetri's primary physical exercise is sex—with women. In his eyes, that's about as masculine as you can get.

> I just feel masculine in the sense that like when I spend time with women, I feel very masculine, and when I spend time with men, I also feel masculine. I feel like one of the boys when I am with women. It's very hard to describe this because it's such a fundamental thing about, like one of the primary drivers for sexual contact.

Demetri's girl crushes began early, starting at age 5. Why this girl? She was "super pretty," and they played together all the time. Demetri has no memory of ever telling her about his feelings. "Definitely not." His parents considered them "cute together."

This crush did not count, however, as Demetri's earliest sexual memory. He struggled with the question, pausing: "This will definitely take me a minute. It's like trying to look at the other side of a wall or something because it's so hard to think like that now." The earliest memory was reserved for a *Playboy* magazine stolen by a friend from his father when both were "my reaction wants to be 10 or 11."

> Definitely at that point, I already had a preconceived notion of what sexuality was. So it must have been before then.
>
> R: Did you tell anyone about the memory?
>
> I don't think it was a specific type of thing that I wanted to keep from people. But I think it was the kind of thing where I just didn't really discuss it with other people because it wasn't something that you would bring up kind of randomly to a friend because you wouldn't know if they would have been exposed to the same thing. It wouldn't be something you brought up to an adult because it wouldn't be appropriate, and that was probably before I really had like intense sexual conceptions about females.

Once the interview moved beyond his childhood, Demetri's memory picked up considerably.

ADOLESCENCE

Demetri's ideas about females were enhanced not only by *Playboy* but also by Internet porn, which he had heard about from his school buddies. They were at the threshold of puberty. Was it helpful to have access to porn at age 11? Demetri has second thoughts about porn as a positive thing.

> Probably if I had to fundamentally say, I would say "bad" just because it's taken time to re-learn, because pornography is so different from actual sexual interaction, and there was definitely a period of re-learning what real sexuality was or like breaking misconceptions about what it would be like. I've thought a lot about what sexuality must have been like for people who had no conception of what it was like before they got married and then somebody was like, "This is what you are supposed to do," and they were like, "Okay." It conditions you to have a specific preference towards something that is commercialized and fake. The audio is very fake, the facial expressions are very fake, and those are the things that form our primary conceptions about things sexually. Definitely gave me some sense of what physical pleasure for both sexes would be, but the thing is those conceptions I had were not completely accurate. They had to be re-learned anyway.

A year later, Demetri's dad tried to have a sex talk with him, but it was too embarrassing, too late, and too religious. Demetri's response was typical: "I already know this. Can you leave? I know. I go to church. I know. And Dad was like, 'Okay.' " The ideal age for a sex talk with his dad would have been two years earlier, according to Demetri, before he discovered pornography. Demetri's aunt reminded him about the church's stance on sex:

> Sex is like a Band-Aid and the more people you stick to it, the less sticky it gets. So if you plan to marry someone and raise children with them and spend a life with them, it's really important that you keep stickiness in your Band-Aid.

Demetri loves this adage, though he's not sure he has a lot of stickiness left.

Without a wet dream, Demetri's first orgasm was "self-inflicted," around age 11, with an assist from Internet porn. It was an excellent experience, but aware of social norms, he shared the thrill of the event with no one.

DATING AND SEX

Demetri turned to dating somewhat earlier than most of his friends, at age 13. He enjoyed the social perks of dating Katrina, though at the time he thought she was more of a "pain in the ass than it was worth." He didn't even particularly enjoy her presence, though Katrina did give him his first kiss; they never made out. Thus began a familiar pattern throughout Demetri's early adolescence before he entered into a long-term relationship in high school, and his first sexual intercourse.

This was not, however, Demetri's first genital contact. Rather, a family visit with friends netted Demetri, age 14, his father's friend's daughter—an "older woman," a year his senior. The story he is about to tell me is accurate, Demetri assured me, because "I kept a journal for like two weeks in my whole life, and it happened to be during this."

> I immediately hit it off with her, and there was an immediate draw towards each other. I had prior girlfriends before then, and I had made out with people but never had that. We went on a hike and were on a cliff and just naturally kind of sat down and then laid down together and then eventually I think I kissed her first, but it really didn't matter at that point. After like four hours of making out, she put her hand down my pants, and I remember really soon after that, we heard her dad screaming because we had been in the woods for so long. It was funny.
>
> I am still very good friends with her. I really, really liked her as a person too, which was the awesome part . . . There was none of the problems of breakup because it was just understood that it couldn't actually happen because we lived on separate sides of large, expansive land . . . I visited her last year, and I had sex with her, too. That was after four years, almost five years.

Demetri rated this experience as "very enjoyable," an 11 on a 10-point scale. Plus, he shared this hookup experience with his guy friends, who were quite happy (jealous?) for him.

His long-term relationship lasted two years, during which Demetri "definitely loved her for a good chunk of that period."

A carefully planned first intercourse was a centerpiece of his high school sophomore year.

We were in drama club together and we were doing a Jekyll and Hyde, and there is a scene in where there is a brothel. Part of the show was that she had to do a striptease for me. There was a lap dance in the brothel. I remember practicing that one day and just being like okay. We had been seeing each other for a month and a half, and then the show ended. We hooked up that night or like the next morning. We exchanged oral sex, and then we started dating, and we were probably dating for two months. I remember thinking that it was an extremely short period of time. But as far as comfort went, it was perfect, so we didn't really mind.

It kind of sucked. It was not really enjoyable for her or me. Not enjoyable for her for classic female not enjoying first sex reasons. Not enjoyable for me because the condoms we got were too small. We didn't realize I would need larger condoms. It was kind of like putting on an extra small glove and trying to do work. It was painful for both of us. It sucked pretty bad. The next time we had sex it was fantastic.

R: Did you tell anyone?

I wanted to respect her privacy. I remember her telling me that she told like one or two friends. So I told one or two of my closest friends. I specifically didn't want to brag. It wasn't like I had achieved something. It was like we had shared something really special, and I wanted to respect that.

R: Was it true love?

I feel like true love is the love that's fundamental in all living things that you share with everything. Like God's love. Not like love you share with another person that is temporary that will die when you die. Like love that was there before you came and will be there after you are gone and after all humans are gone.

They went to separate colleges, and the long-distance relationship faltered, as they typically do at this age. Although they "really, really liked each other, being apart was just killing us so we split up."

SEXUAL AND ROMANTIC STATUS

Demetri wasn't pleased with questions regarding his ideal sexual and romantic self. What he is now is natural and thus what he'll be in the future.

> My issue with this is that I don't really have an ideal orientation. I feel like that's fundamentally lying to yourself. I don't have a future one that I want to be because I just occupy what I am currently and don't particularly put thought or stress into what I should be or what people expect of me. I just do what comes naturally.

R: What are you today?

> I consider myself primarily heterosexual, but I am not really sexually attracted to men. I can appreciate aesthetic beauty of males, but I am not the type of person who will be like, "I will never be attracted to men," because I am attracted to individuals, and if I were to meet a man who I was attracted to, I would not be afraid to be attracted to them. That's currently my life. I definitely am currently heterosexual. As far as future and ideal though, I guess probably in the future I will remain heterosexual, but I don't have an ideal.

Demetri used the words *primarily heterosexual*, but I needed him to clarify this because he selected "exclusively straight" on sexual orientation and "mostly straight" on romantic orientation. Has he ever had a crush on a guy?

> No, I wouldn't say that. Not even strong feelings. I've definitely had moments with guys where I'll put my arm around them and just chill, and it's not like sexual in the way it would be with a female but it does share the fundamental warmth and affection that I would share with a female. They are definitely very distinctly separated. I would describe sexuality as like a twang and a burn. It's more fiery. A romantic relationship is an affectionate warmth. It's soft and dull. I've had both with women but only the affectionate with a guy.

It's likely this "affectionate warmth" that gays pick up on when they come onto Demetri, requiring him to clarify to gay men "plenty of times" his nonexistent sexual intents. However, he is flattered by their attention.

> The first time a guy came onto me was between my junior and senior year of high school. I don't separate male taste in men from female taste in men as far as what they are looking for. It's like, "Oh, cool, someone is attracted to me." I remember the first time being like, "Oh, you know, this hasn't happened to me before. I will give you a chance." I started going in towards them, and the type of energy I felt was not what I was looking for. It felt not right, and I was like, "Whoa, I don't think this is not right fundamentally. I am fine with this. But for me this just doesn't work." The feeling is like sinking and kind of twisting.

R: What would you do today if this happened to you?

> It still does happen, pretty frequently. I am still usually flattered. Then I try as nice as a way as possible. Like, if I'm dancing on a dance floor I will try to get up next to the guy so I can say something to him without other people hearing it like, "Even though you are really good looking, I am not into you but don't be put off but if I was, I would totally be down." I always try to be really nice about it, and usually people leave smiling.

Demetri clearly has no problem with gay people, in part because Costa, an older brother (he has three), has bisexual interests. "He experimented in college or high school, but now he seems primarily straight." Demetri believes men are designed to have a good time with sex, regardless if they're into women or men. His entire family is "ultra-liberal," and he gave himself a 9 on a 10-point scale of conservative to liberal.

Demetri is more of a romantic than a sex machine—a 7 out of 10 (he loves to invent 10-point scales). He explained that he's "not a scumbag when I hook up with people." He respects women as persons and cares for their happiness. "I get a bigger kick about other people having a good time."

R: How do you see your future?

> I don't right now actually. I've been with a girl here for like two years . . . I met her the summer I was first here and hit it off with

her. We were very close, and we kept in touch when I was in my
senior year of high school even though she was like a college
sophomore, which was kind of funny to me.

Demetri doubts he'll marry her, or anyone. He feels perhaps a
long-term girlfriend is best. For now, Demetri is focused on his
science career.

MUSINGS

In most respects, Demetri's developmental history is prototypically
heterosexual. He's within the mainstream range of masculinity:
he had male friends as a child, developed girl crushes, watched
porn around pubertal onset, and experienced his first masturbation around that time. He's a deep thinker with his own take
on life. Sexually, Demetri is an earlier player than his male peers
across the board in terms of his first date, genital contact, engaging in intercourse, and developing a relationship. His first experience with sexual intercourse wasn't great, his parents didn't
have an on-time sex talk with him, and he used porn for sex
education—all fairly typical of the straight guys I interviewed.

Although he is into both sex and romance with women,
Demetri is a self-described romantic. He loves women and anticipates continuing to be in a long-term relationship with a woman,
yet his romantic side is something other than totally straight. Gay
guys pursue Demetri as a prospect, misinterpreting his romantic attraction to guys as sexual interest. I detected no evidence Demetri
shares their sexual desires—though he turns them down in a nice,
thoughtful way. He's flattered, which has less to do with sexuality
than with being told he's attractive and, more importantly, evoking
his same-sex romantic self.

It's intriguing that Demetri (also see Ryan and Kyle) has
three older brothers, with a six-year gap between him and Costa,
his "bisexual experimenting" brother. Given that he has no known
genetic kin who is gay, Demetri's family pattern of male births
fits the *older brother hypothesis*—increasing same-sex sexuality
with each successive male pregnancy. That is, perhaps the maternal immune response to having multiple male fetuses (large
gaps in between live births suggests possible failed pregnancies

and thus potentially additional male fetuses) was not sufficient to produce a full-fledged gay boy but was adequate to create (as the two youngest boys) slightly nonheterosexual sons (see Appendix B). Demetri should thank his older brothers for his ever so slight same-sex romantic orientation—either biologically or for modeling mostly heterosexuality. Either one might work.

ricky

*It's more like, "I want to be that big," rather than,
"Oh, I want to do stuff with him."* (RICKY, AGE 22)

RICKY REPORTED low levels of sexual and romantic interest in
guys, raising the question of whether his level is typical of straight
guys. I'm uncertain how critical it is, but it's worth noting that
Ricky was a late developer in terms of puberty. Though he appears
to have been exceedingly drawn to girls and women throughout
his life, his genital fascination with them was considerably lower
than that of many other boys. However, a parallel interest in guys
did not divert his heterosexuality. Although I have insufficient
information, my best guess is that Ricky's limited homoeroticism
(appreciation of hot guys, admiring large penises, making out with
a guy on a dare) might be more of a reflection on other aspects of
his sexuality.

THE INTERVIEW

Ricky, age 22, called to say he was running a half-hour late, and
he apologized. Slightly shorter than the average guy, with jet-

black hair and a slightly messy appearance, Ricky possessed an informality in his demeanor. He wore baggy shorts, a T-shirt, and flip-flops, and he has several colorful tattoos. Extremely friendly with a killer smile, Ricky was happy to do the interview, initially for the money—each interviewee received a small amount of money for his participation—and afterward he realized he liked telling his story. Heavily involved in technology research throughout his college career, Ricky intends to use his knowledge to improve the physical and mental health of children. An unapologetic Eagle Scout, Ricky is a fraternity member, sings in an a cappella group, and participates in snowboarding competitions. How do these fit together? Ricky shrugged.

The interview was longer than most because Ricky struggled with his memory and paused frequently, deep in thought. He nearly always retrieved a memory and then apologized for his memory lapses. He attributed his uncertainties about the particulars of his life to stress. He was nearing graduation from college but had no job lined up. In a follow-up phone interview two years later, Ricky had found his job but was no better at accessing his memory during our conversation.

CHILDHOOD

As a kid, Ricky did the usual kid stuff—Pop Warner football, soccer, and swimming, which were his main sports. In college, it was golf, cycling, volleyball, and intermural basketball. All his best friends were other boys; when asked to rate his masculinity on a scale from 1 to 10, Ricky gave himself a 7, maybe an 8. "I have pretty man-wired thinking." He's competitive and wants to take charge of situations. His self-described femininity is manifested, he said, in an inability to dissociate sex and love. Unlike the "macho men" in his fraternity, Ricky is selective in who he hooks up with.

Despite his poor memory, Ricky vividly and with considerable passion recalled his earliest sex memory. This will turn out to be a key feature of his sexuality—a fact I only realized at the end of the interview.

> I used to have a lot of female friends growing up, which is kind of the side effect of me having a pink parka when I was playing

in the snow one time and made female friends who thought I was a girl. That's a separate story. We used to play these games when I was like 4 or 5 or 6 that was like you would be pretending to be a dog or something like that. Kind of like *101 Dalmatians* like the poacher would take you and put you in a trap and the other dogs would have to come and save you and things like that. It [would] pretty much always be that I did the saving. I don't know if that was me being the man in the group or something like that, but we would always tie each other up. We would be downstairs in the basement tied to the pole with like a jump rope or something, and I remember that I had dreams when I was younger with, I explicitly remember the image of life-size Barbie dolls. One of those tied to a pole in my basement, and that was my first sexual arousing memory. I don't know if I had started kindergarten or not.

In third grade, Ricky began having secret crushes. His first crush was Carrie with freckles, one of the popular girls who responded to his overtures by chastising him for the brand of shoes he was wearing. His second crush resulted from snooping. Ricky seized a chance to read the diary of Cathy, a very popular girl. Seeing "Ricky" circled with a heart, Ricky told her how much he too loved her. He was the wrong Ricky.

ADOLESCENCE

Puberty also wasn't so great for Ricky since he was a late bloomer. His physical budding began during his freshman year of high school. In trying to remember when and how he learned about puberty and the mechanics of sex, Ricky listed sixth grade as drug education, seventh as health class, and eighth as sex education—or was it ninth? One important topic covered was wet dreams. Previously when he heard a boy report a wet dream, "I thought that the person had peed the bed, and I was like, 'Ha-ha, they peed the bed.'" Sex education was also useful in teaching him to never have sex without a condom. Since then, "I always tried to practice things safely."

By the time his parents discussed sex with him, Ricky told them he already knew everything, "So we don't have to talk about this." When I asked why the sex talk wasn't earlier, Ricky excused them as "busy people."

> I don't think they were afraid of having the talk. It was just kind of like they were always busy people and busy with school, and I had a lot of extracurricular and stuff like that. The time we spent together was fun times over dinner and vacations, hanging. It just never really came up. It was just kind of like, I don't know if ever there really was a serious time to talk. I couldn't give an exact answer for that . . .
>
> I don't think I ever talked with them. So, sophomore year, I had a steady girlfriend. My first steady girlfriend and we never had sex, but we did oral sex and I guess digital hand sex. But I never really brought any of that up with my parents. I don't feel the need to talk with them about that.

An earlier conversation might have prevented Ricky from believing his first orgasm, from a wet dream, was peeing in bed. "Jeez, I couldn't remember specifically, probably sometime in early high school." It turned out to be a slightly negative experience because he felt out of control of his body. "The general protocol is take off your underwear, put the underwear in the hamper, put on new underwear, and nobody asked questions."

Sophomore year Ricky began masturbating. He searched for porn on the Internet and masturbated to his preferred erotic images. Unfortunately, he didn't know about clearing his browsing history on the family's computer and thus received an embarrassing lecture from his parents.

> I already knew what I wanted to look for was "Girl tied to bed." It wasn't like I watched these images and started thinking like, "Oh now I want to do this sort of sexually deviant behavior." I guess that's kind of telling that I call it deviant behavior.
>
> My parents gave me a lecture about how those girls didn't grow up with good families and things like that. I guess the first image I remember was a woman tied to a bed. Full hands and feet. The first time I masturbated was in the shower. I had some soap and figured this was what you were supposed to do, rub in and out with your hand. I did what felt good.

It did feel good, but Ricky "definitely did not, certainly didn't, for sure didn't tell anyone." He didn't think others needed to know what he was doing. His parents, however, caught on. "They would come and like knock on the door every once in a while because I would be spending a lot of time showering. I do in general like long showers, without masturbating." He soon had another source for orgasms.

DATING AND SEX

Although a late bloomer physically, by his sophomore year of high school Ricky had a steady girlfriend, Gabriella, with wandering hands and a desire for oral sex. His parents knew the two were dating but not that they were sexually active.

> I guess it was a couple months of making out and we went for a walk in the park, and that was the first time she touched my penis, and then later I snuck out of my house and walked two miles to meet up with her when she was at a friend's sleeping over. We met up outside, and that was the first time I had oral sex.
>
> She took the initiative, but neither of us had an orgasm, at least I don't think she did, to my knowledge. It was kind of weird. I wasn't initiating anything, so it was kind of bizarre for me. She offered to have sex with me one time when she was at a friend's house sleeping over, and I had left and walked over, and I didn't go along with it. I guess it's kind of a similar thing for the first time that she went in my pants and everything. I was nervous about it. I would rate it as a slightly shaded negative [experience]. I mean obviously not horribly negative because we were making out and that was kind of good, but I don't know if I was quite ready for that.

They soon established a routine—a movie downstairs, make out on the couch, and oral or hand sex. One day, however, Ricky's dad came down looking for his golf magazines: "We stopped, and he walked back upstairs, and a couple minutes later the dog came down. A couple minutes later he was like, 'What are you guys doing down there?' And I was like, 'Oh we're just hanging out.'" He asked Ricky to take the dog for a walk.

The relationship with Gabriella lasted about six months, and as it progressed Ricky became "really nervous if my penis was big enough and if it had been different from the ones she had seen before or anything like that." Both were virgins, but she wanted to have intercourse before Ricky did, which was the primary reason for the breakup. "I wasn't ready for that and she wanted to, so she went on to someone else who was willing to provide that."

After Gabriella, a senior named Kristen, a swim teammate, came into Ricky's life, and they dated for two years. Kristen initiated the first kiss on the team bus, motivated by Ricky's goofy glasses and hat, which made him look "different or sexy." Later during a discussion on favorite milkshakes Kristen invited Ricky over for a movie and a "special milkshake." I'm abbreviating this rather lengthy, detailed narrative.

> We go over, and eventually something happens in the movie we are watching, and we get into an argument about it, and we are arguing back and forth, and our faces get close, and we finally kissed. I know it's not what you asked about, but I am glad I remembered for my own well-being. We were doing that for a little while and after a couple of these date things I was sitting in the car and I was like, "What is going on here? What is our situation? Are we dating are we not dating?" And she was like, "Well, I don't know," and eventually we decided that we were going to date. Wonderful! I think that was only a two-week period of time that we were in the gray zone.
>
> Then we were dating, and we were exclusive, and around finals for that period of time we had half days and our parents didn't have half days. We went to her house, and the first couple days it was more of the same. Oral sex for the first time was after prom, my junior year her senior year . . . After a couple days, I think I brought it up at one point. I rode my bike to the store and bought my first box of condoms. I couldn't even drive yet! I was 16 years old. I guess we had sex during one of those half days during the exam period.
>
> I brought it up the first time, and she said she wasn't ready. And then a couple days later, she initiated having sex.

The first time was "kind of awkward because I knew it was hurting her, and we had to try a couple different positions before something could work right. But we kept at it, and eventually it got a lot better." Ricky had an orgasm and Kristen didn't. Ricky shared his new status of getting over a "barrier," with his best friend, who laughed.

The two lasted through Ricky's freshman year in college as a long-distance relationship. Though the love they shared was certainly the strongest Ricky had ever felt and the relationship was meaningful and serious, "I don't think it was the true love, forever type." Ricky has been single since then, though flirting and searching for the right woman.

Considering his future, I asked Ricky about his preference for a romantic relationship (which for him must be monogamous) versus "chalking up the numbers."

> I am actively searching around for somebody who is special. So I am looking for someone. I have been single for a couple years now. Somebody I can be in a relationship with. Until then, I am just kind of test-driving a couple different models before I can find the one for me, I guess. I feel like it's an important skill, not just like chalking up the numbers. But when I run into the girl who is going to make me really happy I want to have the skill set that is necessary in order for her to be attracted to me and know that I can confidently go forward and get her to be attracted to me. It's kind of like, well, I have to get my practice in. I like talking to girls and flirting is really fun, and I mean I would like to have sex with a lot of girls if that is an option. I think eventually I would be. If someone came around right now who was really special and interesting to me and wasn't taken the way they always are, I would be willing to be a serious relationship.
>
> I definitely want to get married and have kids and a family. Things like that. I want to be married to a girl I love. I want to be married in my early 30s, hopefully not late 30s. I want to have fun in my 20s.

SEXUAL AND ROMANTIC STATUS

After this display of heterosexuality, I ask, consistent with my interview protocol, whether he's had crushes on guys. Ricky didn't think so, and was then more definite.

There has never been any sort of romantic attraction. I have had a lot of really close male friends that I would do anything for.

R: What's the difference between the crushes you've had on girls and the intense guy friends?

I feel like guy friends are more like allies and a lover is more of someone who is part of you. I feel like it's more intense with love. There is obviously the sex component as well. I could never see myself having sex with a guy or any of my male friends. I could appreciate a good-looking male guy. Like, "Hey that guy is pretty hot," but it's more like, "I want to be that big," rather than "Oh, I want to do stuff with him." I feel like male relationships are kind of like, "You do your thing and I'll do my thing, and you know I got your back if you need each other." But I feel like a male-female relationship is more intertwined with your personal life and stuff.

R: Have you ever had a guy come on to you?

I don't recall specifically.

R: What would you do?

I would probably do the same thing if a girl came on to me. I would laugh a little bit and change the conversation topic and probably go and do something else.

Ricky once made out with a guy as a dare. After drinking, Ricky wanted a cigarette, and in return the guy asked him to make out. For Ricky, this wasn't a manifest sexual or romantic intent.

Consistent with others in his generation, Ricky is "pretty welcoming" of gay people, and he supports marriage equality. By virtue of being younger than his parents and around gay and bisexual people at college, Ricky believes he's more gay positive than they are, though his father has lots of gay friends and a gay nephew.

At the close of the interview, we discussed Ricky's first sexual memory and what he found by Google for his first masturbation—girl tied to bed.

R: What is the meaning of this for your life?

I guess it was kind of a stigma associated with bondage and things like that which is actually something that I am kind of into, and I think might be a result of this early memory and the games that we played together. So I am more reluctant to volunteer that information. But I don't know about if at the time I was less reluctant to volunteer. I was 5 years old. I didn't know it was, that was a weird thing. I don't remember specifically telling anyone about it.

R: Do you think this has meaning for you?

Maybe it's a preference that I have always had and as a result of that, this was particularly interesting. But I don't know. I can vividly remember this. Especially the dream about the life-sized Barbie doll tied to [a] pole and things like that. I guess it could have had an impact on my life or in my future sexual interests and things like that . . . I don't know what it is. It is what it is.

MUSINGS

The question I grappled with is whether Ricky belongs in this book. His professed homoeroticism is quite low, perhaps consistent with straight guys. Ricky's intense guy friendships are frequently shared by other straight men, he's into sports, and he has dated and had sex with girls/women. He expressly stated he has few romantic desires for guys and doesn't want to date them. Ricky appears to be exclusively straight when it comes to his romantic self.

But what about his sexual self—is he typical of a straight guy? He confesses to admiring hot guys and large penises, and he made out with a guy on a dare; yet his desire for male sexual contact is minimal. Should these homoerotic aspects be discounted because they are not uncommon among straight guys? I'm not sure how common they indeed are.

I include Ricky here because of his unique sexuality—which might place him on the asexual end of the sexual spectrum. His admission to having a low sex drive, revealed in his masturbation ("I masturbate less than most of my friends. I give it lower priority.") is one indication. A second is his lack of heterosexual sex, which Ricky views as primarily necessary to maintain a relationship. But how does his homoeroticism fit in with his asexuality?

One possibility is that Ricky's hypothesized asexuality and homoeroticism are secondary to his keener interest in erotic practices and sexualized power-role-playing that include elements of bondage/discipline, dominance/submission, and sado-masochism among consensual participants. These interests have been present in Ricky's life since an early age (being tied up, rescuing Barbie) and continued through early adolescence ("girl tied to bed" kink-typed porn) into the present (being in control, taking charge). Within this context, the gender of the other person(s) might have less meaning than the actual activities.

If Ricky were to have sexual contact with guys, my best guess is that it would only occur within such activities, perhaps motivated by his kink-oriented porn watching. Ricky might not be exclusively straight in the context of the kink world.

chris

[I'm] pretty sure [that] I'm going toward female attractions and am questioning my attraction with guy friends. (CHRIS, AGE 20)

OUR THIRD PRIMARILY STRAIGHT YOUNG MAN, Chris, blurs the most lines among exclusively, primarily, and mostly straight sexual and romantic orientations. Each could claim Chris. His homoeroticism is clearly present, but is it unusually high for a straight man? Although Chris has never had sex or dated a guy, he has considered having sex with a guy, and his intense guy friendships border on infatuations. Pondering these patterns, Chris concluded that as best as he can determine, he's *pretty sure* he's straight—but only, he claims, because of how he was raised.

THE INTERVIEW

His girlfriend, a "serious candidate" for a future wife, referred Chris, age 20, to the interview, though Chris claimed he had also seen posters around campus and was going to volunteer. My first impression of Chris had him pegged as a classic Pacific beach skater, but without the skateboard. Immediately charming and radiating warmth, slight of build, two-toned short hair (blond on top, dark brown on the sides), sloppy shorts embedded with a sunset and an ocean, several long-sleeved T-shirts, and an accent I couldn't place, Chris had a firm handshake, made prolonged eye contact, and moved his chair closer to me. Given his easygoing, casual look, I was taken aback when Chris said his professional goal is marketing or advertising—but then he added with "a social justice bent."

It was not an easy interview—Chris began asking me questions midway through the interview, such as "What do you think I should do?," so I continually needed to redirect him back to the standard protocol. He would relent, at least until the next issue that piqued his interest. His quest for knowledge was endearing, though a bit frustrating in terms of completing the task at hand of recording his life story. We didn't linger long on his childhood years because Chris didn't remember it as a cheerful time. "I wasn't a happy kid." All of that changed when he connected with adolescent friends.

CHILDHOOD

During his early years, Chris was interested in sci-fi fantasy, *Star Trek,* and soccer in conjunction with a group of like-minded boys. "We did weird things and imaginary games, convincing ourselves that there really was an imaginary world that was real, that there were ghosts to fight. Really crazy stuff. Broke me out of my comfort zone." Chris wanted everyone to like him, and he detested fighting, either verbally or physically. His claim to childhood fame was "the guy who fainted" in school ("but only once"). Chris also played with Pokémon cards, something he believed to be uncool.

His first girl crush was prepuberty, in sixth grade, because the girl "was pretty, played sports, and was different from other girls because she was willing to hang out with us boys." Plus she played tetherball and was good at it. Did he tell her about his crush? "No way," he said. But it did provide confidence that at least he could talk to girls.

Chris considers himself masculine because "I have a girl-friend, lots of male friends, enjoy sports, am competitive, and sometimes grow out my beard. I am not a big guy, but I am loud sometimes." He has no desire to be more or less masculine.

ADOLESCENCE

Everything changed for Chris in seventh grade when his parents enrolled him in a private all-boys Catholic school. He lost his old friends and then slowly found other boys, with whom he played soccer. The friendships were sufficiently strong that even today all six remain best friends. "This is kind of dumb," he warned me, but during Boy Scout campfires, "we had deep existential conversations, especially when relatives started to die, and [we did] weird stuff like catch a grasshopper and put it on an ant hill and watch them eat it." Together the friends went through a spiritual adventure that changed Chris's perspective on the world. They asked lots of questions, pondered, and were "thinkers" (note at this point of the interview Chris began asking me questions). Chris thought of himself as "elite, better than most, and it allowed me to go through a spiritual adventure and increased my perspective on the world." Chris got religion and converted to a mystical form of Buddhism while at Catholic school.

When Chris returns home from college to the West Coast, his friends pick him up at the airport; then they party and dominate his time, causing Chris's parents to complain they never get to see him anymore. These friendships are "like another family." They are the antidote to Chris's feelings of isolation and lack of confidence because they "are accepting with lots of concepts, open to people, thinkers, and easy to get along with." In particular, his best friend is an adventurous West Coast type, who is relaxed, mooches off the system, and "made me work really hard, and this is why I'm here today."

Puberty, most evident to Chris from his increased body hair, "hit me between 13 and 15, like hit it later than most of my peers." Once it arrived, Chris was pleased because he had his first wet dream, though he can't remember the featured female star who inspired it. Rare among boys, he told his parents—in large part because "I was proud of myself for maturing, I guess. They were laughing at me in a joking manner. I announced to them, 'I'm a man now.' "

His next sexual accomplishment waited until sophomore year when Chris "finally succeeded" in masturbating. His mind's eye was focused on girls, and he was "pretty happy I finally could do it and I didn't tell anyone initially. It wasn't a big deal at all." Although he had sex education in sixth grade (before Catholic school), he learned about sex mostly from his friends. Nevertheless, his parents followed up the class with a birds-and-bees talk. "Sex was not a taboo topic in my home." Chris's response was, "Come on guys I know this." They ignored his plea and told Chris how to use a condom. As a prepubertal sixth grader, Chris dismissed the information because he wasn't yet interested in sex.

DATING AND SEX

Attending a Catholic school, enjoying intense boy friendships, and having a late onset of puberty did not strongly encourage Chris to try early dating or sex with girls. Though an all-girls school existed right across the street, "the nuns kept a tight control on the girls." Indeed, it was not until his sophomore year of high school that Chris even wanted to date.

His first romantic relationship and first sexual contact also waited until sophomore year—not of high school but college—both with his girlfriend at the time. He entered college sexually inexperienced but highly motivated.

> We were dating for three weeks and it was, I guess you'd call it, mutual masturbation. We had a conversation about how far we'd go. Both had orgasms. She had one prior sexual experience but with no orgasm. It was very awkward and then very relaxed after the first time. It continued because the relationship was working so well we were willing to risk investing in it and both agreed it was a good idea.
>
> Two months later we decided to do it [intercourse] after the "I love you" stage. I was hesitant and had thought I wouldn't do it, but the hormones got the better of me. It was not good because I caused pain when I broke her hymen. We both expected that it wouldn't be good.

Compared to many young men of his generation, Chris's sexual and romantic repertoire remains limited.

SEXUAL AND ROMANTIC STATUS

Given the intensity of his male friendships, I asked Chris if he had or wanted to have sexual interactions with males.

> No. I thought about it with a really good male friend, but I never saw myself doing it. My high school was known as having gays, and this was perceived as very negative. So I had lots of gay friends, and we'd talk about what it was like. I was attracted to these guys. I really thought about it but couldn't feel it as with a girl. Now I'm even more radicalized because I'm with a girl . . .
>
> There were no rumors about my sexuality in senior high. Pretty sure I'm going toward female attractions and am questioning my attraction with guy friends. In college, pretty sure it is female attractions.

This sounded just a little iffy to me, which motivated some follow-up questions.

> R: Ideally, what would you like your sexuality to be?
>
> I'm good with the status quo, and if I change my mind I won't be upset.
>
> R: Can you change your sexuality?
>
> [It's a] born ability. I don't know, but more nature than nurture with some more likely to be gay. Why me? Don't know. It [heterosexuality] could have been pushed on me. No decision on my part. I was born where I was and in a relationship with a girl makes me more heterosexual because it is what I'm used to.
>
> R: Where are you on the Kinsey scale?
>
> [After many questions on Kinsey's theory and research, Chris concluded,] Don't know where I am on the spectrum but close to a Kinsey 0.

Chris admitted to being slightly homophobic, though he tries hard not to be. "In some cases, a tiny bit, not with people I know but [I feel a] slight uneasiness with gay guys, but I don't want to hurt anyone's feelings. It is unfair to treat people as a group. I'm myself have been marginalized [via his Buddhism]. It was very powerful, and I don't want anyone to feel that way."

MUSINGS

On the questionnaire tracking his sexual and romantic develop-ment, Chris indicated that he had no attraction to men. What-ever his sexuality and romantic inclinations, Chris is fine with it. The intriguing aspect is that, despite his 100 percent sexual attraction to women, Chris is not in complete closure regarding his heterosexuality. He's only "pretty sure" about his attractions to women, and he's "*close* to a Kinsey 0."

Chris has thought about having sex with a guy, but he hasn't pursued it because it doesn't quite feel right. Or did he not go there because, as he says, he's slightly homophobic? Yet Chris is certainly not hesitant to tell his male friends that he loves them, and they hug on sight. One of the advantages to being gay, according to Chris, is a guy "wouldn't have to go outside of the same-sex group" for sex. Is he referring to this long-standing intense friendship group?

Do these indicate a slight degree of homoeroticism? Per-haps Chris is in between straight and mostly straight—it's a close call. Statements about his sexual and romantic self are indicative of his being incredibly sexually and romantically fluid, leaving doors open, willing to consider all options, and being exception-ally honest with himself. I'm not sure, but I'll split the difference and give Chris a Kinsey 0.5 score.

progressive mostly straight

*[It's] just wrong to go against someone
because of their sexual orientation.* (DILLON, AGE 20)

ALTHOUGH MOSTLY STRAIGHT MEN'S EROTIC and romantic
attractions to males are likely hardwired, probably due to genetics
or prenatal hormones, it's not true for all of them. Some young
men identify as mostly straight not because of their biology but
because of their progressive nature, attitudes, and values. These
progressive mostly straight youths are our focus in this chapter.

It proved to be challenging, if not problematic, to place these
young men on the spectrum. Some identified as mostly straight
on their online survey but elsewhere, including in the interview,
expressed little or no sexual or romantic interest in males. Why
this contradictory pattern? Whether such young men are truly
mostly straight grew into a matter of internal debate for me.
Then I realized the pattern they had in common: decidedly left-
leaning social, philosophical, political, even radical propensities
coupled with positive and abundant personal experiences with
gay people while growing up.

None felt constrained by traditional notions of heterosexuality and, indeed, they detested them. They had no fear that they might be perceived as gay—in fact, they rather enjoyed the gay assumption. They hugged male friends, politically defended gay rights, and were not offended if gay guys hit on them. They rejected what they viewed as the regressive attitudes and sexual prejudices of earlier generations—especially those of their parents' generation—and were frequently willing to fight for their elimination through political action. They loved living on the new frontier of sexuality and were not afraid to align themselves with their gay brothers and sisters, politically and socially. One young man raised money for people with AIDS in Africa. Another sang in a gay chorus. Another marched as an ally in a gay pride parade. Another encouraged his like-minded friends to proudly "come out" as *queer,* as he himself had.

During their interviews, the progressive mostly straight youths rejected any attempts to place them into a rigid sexual identity box. Yes, we're straight, they said, but why should we restrict our identities—or, for that matter, anyone's sexuality— to archaic straight-and-narrow categories? They reveled in their ability to withstand social scrutiny and professed little concern about what others thought about their sexuality.

This revolutionary perspective did not, however, change their own sexual and romantic inclinations. Their degree of same-sex sexuality was usually quite small: around 5 percent of their attractions, fantasies, and/or crushes. None had had genital contact or romantic relations with a male, and none had any intent ever having any.

- "Something that never crossed my mind. I had friends who dated guys but never an interest of mine."
- "Everyone has a gay thought that a male is attractive, but it's not for me. I prefer where I'm at."
- "Never interested to explore male sexuality. Always comfortable in my own sexuality."

At this point, I found myself puzzled. These statements are what I might have expected from a progressive straight guy. But these young men self-reported that they are mostly straight even though all had the clear option of declaring themselves exclusively straight. What did they mean? They had minimal same-sex attractions and were uninterested in, had no desire for, and had no thoughts about sexual or romantic interactions with guys. Why did they say they had a degree of same-sex sexuality? Here are several quotable clues that might explain their response.

- "A woman mentor to me through elementary school is gay, so [I was] introduced [to it] at an early age. Never saw it as bad or isolating thing. Just transition to the normal world."
- "My upbringing doesn't consider it strange. It is another way or style of life that is okay with me. Not fair to gays to judge them in certain ways. I do have gay friends."
- "In high school one of my best friends, a year younger, came out to me as bisexual and was dating a guy. We did sports together."
- "My girlfriend is bisexual, and we've had long conversations about sexuality . . . [I've met] a range of people of all sexual orientations."
- "I'm comfortable with my sexuality. I have a girlfriend, and there have been guys who made advances on me and I said, 'No,' and they said they regretted that. I have good friends who are gay."
- "Gay males are more sensitive, and straight males are insensitive."

We know that one of the best predictors of acceptance and support of gay people is to know someone close, usually a friend or relative, who is gay. These same individuals usually believe that sexual orientation, regardless of the specific sexuality, is hardwired and thus not a matter of choice. The progressive mostly straight youths generally followed a social constructionist perspective regarding sexuality, gender differences, and life in general, so they doubted or were dismissive of the biology of sexuality. They simply viewed gayness as a variation along a continuum, which did not, however, imply that people choose their sexuality.

In terms of personal contact, whether a teacher, family member, girlfriend, or friend, all the progressive mostly straight young men know someone close to them who is gay—a friend or someone who came out to them as a matter of personal trust. "I'm a good person to go to because I'm a listener. I inquired about it and what led him to it. Didn't affect my relationship with him." For those who had not yet been the recipient of a coming-out disclosure, they were looking forward to it and expected it soon. "Two friends are possibly gay, and I have my suspicions. I would not stop being their friend, not at all." Quite incredibly, all said they have "no gay fear" and thus have no problems with male intimacy or making recommendations on dress or appearance: "No hang ups, don't worry if I look gay." Another said, "I don't worry about the gay thing. I know I'm not gay, and if I was it would not be an issue."

I had one more test question: "If you discovered you had a gay roommate when you were assigned a dorm room your freshman year, what would you have done?" The answers were consistent: "Not a problem," "Great," and "Whatever." No one would have requested a room change because "I learn from different people." One young man had in fact been assigned a gay roommate in his freshman year of college. "Not a big deal. Genuine person, nice, openly gay and never a subject of any discomfort." He could easily undress in front of his roommate and make accommodations about who had the room on "special" occasions.

The progressive mostly straight young men struck me as the epitome of gay acceptance. They vehemently denied being homophobic and claimed sexual prejudice is a rather stupid thing. Gays are to be admired, they said. "They're scrutinized, lots of pressure, judged more than if straight when applying for jobs. [It] takes strength to be gay."

I can't confirm or deny whether these young men have a slight degree of same-sex sexuality. Nevertheless, they insisted that they were not exclusively straight. I can't tell whether this was a way to align themselves with a perceived oppressed group as a means to signify their solidarity with gays or to claim membership in an edgy sexual culture. My guess is that many of these young men will return to a straight identification over time. All had next to zero interest in pursuing same-sex interests, and all appeared fairly committed to their sexual and romantic alliances with women. If the "right" guy came along would they change their minds? I doubt it.

it's about the sex

I mean, come on, tell me some guys aren't hot!
(MOSTLY STRAIGHT YOUTH, AGE 19)

A YOUTH MIGHT IDENTIFY AS MOSTLY STRAIGHT because he can't deny that some guys are admirably physically and sexually attractive. One interviewee appeared somewhat defensive when he exclaimed, "I mean, come on, tell me some guys aren't hot!" If a guy finds himself staring at other guys in the gym, on the sports field, around the neighborhood, and in *Maxim, Details,* and *Vman,* then how can he say to himself or others that he's totally straight? He notices guys in the buff, and guys who are buff—visually appealing and a pleasure to be around. But this doesn't apply to all men, only some of them, which causes him to wonder what he desires—the toned body, stylistic appearance, athletic ability, muscularity, impressive penis? Or a mostly straight sexuality?

At some point in his developmental history he challenges himself if his interest in the male body means something special. He can't be totally straight, he reasons, because if girls find a guy physically attractive and will have sex with him, then physical attraction=sexual attraction. However, he hedges a bit because he's not quite sure if this equation is universal or applies to him. His same-sex attractions are also apparent when the occasional male pops up in his sexual dreams or masturbatory fantasies. The male's appearance doesn't decrease—and may even increase—the erotic tone of his imagination.

These realizations are the basis for his self-questioning. *Am I really totally straight if I notice attractive guys?* Though he might assume during childhood and early adolescence that his male friends also find other males attractive, they never speak about it. By late adolescence, however, he realizes that other straight men do not share his assessment of other guys. Perhaps, he deduces, like Dillon, that he is merely metrosexual in appearance, fashion, and interpersonal relationships and this extends to his sexuality. Identifying as mostly straight fits this pattern.

He might also recognize that within his limited degree of same-sex attraction is a will and a desire to engage in sexual activities with other males—and perhaps he has done so. It's never been his top priority, and, when given the choice, he will nearly always pursue girls. Although he seldom or never has plans to have sex with a guy, unlike his straight brothers he's not averse to it. He might agree to a three-way or group sex (with another male present) perhaps to entice a girl, though he'd rather have a three-way with two girls and himself. Women are his primary source of sexual desires and fantasies, and he intends to eventually devote his life to one, or several.

Yet neither are mostly straight men willing to rule out future sexual relations with guys to further the experiment or satisfy their curiosity. Nearly all expressed curiosity about what it would be like to have sex with a guy. They're not repulsed by the thought of guys getting it on. Instead, they say "let it be" or "looks interesting." Their willingness to experiment is contingent on both (or more) partners realizing that the goal is sexual pleasure with no strings attached, without meaning. It's what good friends sometimes do when sufficiently horny or when a guy wants to bond with "my buds." Hey, an orgasm is an orgasm! Anything is possible, given the right context with the right person or under the right conditions, though what those circumstances are isn't always clear. At the very least, these thoughts are an expression of his sexual fluidity.

The expressed desire for sexual activities is usually restricted to receptive oral sex or mutual rubbing or showing. Anal intercourse usually feels "too gay," except perhaps if he is the inserter. The mostly straight young man who engages in male-male sexual interactions rarely finds it loathsome or unappealing but rather pleasurable and satisfying for his curiosity. It just isn't his primary focus, and he usually evaluates it as less significant than (though an acceptable and maybe even good substitute for) sex with girls. And it might happen again, especially if girls are involved.

In the next chapter I present vignettes from five mostly straight young men, who may or may not have had limited same-sex genital contact, but have same-sex attractions and some amount of desire for future possibilities.

five young men

WILL

*We'd do sleepovers and rubbing against each other with clothes on,
and we showed each other our genitals.* (WILL, AGE 26)

A 26-year-old graduate student in the humanities, Will came an hour early for the interview and spoke slowly as he twisted the many silver rings on his fingers. Nose piercings, tattoos, and large-framed square glasses completed his look. In his responses, Will was deliberate and thoughtful.

He recalled a typical childhood, "except my parents divorced when I was 2." Neither particularly popular nor an outsider, Will had a small group of male friends who hung out together after school playing football and sledding. Otherwise, he described himself as happy to go to school to be with others and escape his loneliness—happy at least until his friend's brother was violently killed, which profoundly shook him up in terms of what life was all about.

In high school, Will participated in cross-country running and band, and he went to movies, always by himself. He described himself as a fairly assertive and aggressive adolescent, except around girls. He has always been passive about initiating conversation with members of the opposite sex. He wasn't sure "what I wanted from them, but I don't feel that way anymore."

Titillated by showering with his mother when he was 3 years old and seeing Sally Jessy Raphael on television when he was 8, Will began sexually exploring himself soon thereafter. He tried to recall when puberty began for him, but all he could remember was armpit hair. He never had a wet dream though he was close several times before waking, and he could not recall which one of his masturbations was the first. His dad gave him the sex talk in sixth grade, but he learned more by spying on his father and his new girlfriend during their rather frequent sexual escapades.

During middle school, when Will was 12, he and his best friend wrestled a lot, talked about girls, "like Cindy Crawford, and it was sexualized between us. Only guy I had that with. We'd do sleepovers and rubbing against each other with clothes on, and we showed each other our genitals." Although they found it physically gratifying, neither had an orgasm because they were too young. It happened three times.

Will recalled early and frequent girl crushes, with dating following soon thereafter. His first sex with a girlfriend came late, at age 18, and it became a five-year relationship. They had frequent oral (her choice) and vaginal (his choice) sex. This was a young woman who "orgasmed if I touched her." Will claimed to "not really be attracted to guys," then added, after a moment, "for the most part. It would easier if I was gay because I'd have more sex." His current girlfriend has encouraged him to explore his gay nature. When he's with her, he admits, "I can look at guys the way she does." It's not every guy, Will emphasized, only a few.

On the follow-up questionnaire, slightly over a year later, Will reported that he had begun writing poetry and, though he and his girlfriend live far apart, they Skype to enjoy their sexual fantasies with each other. Will intends to have a monogamous, romantic relationship with his current girlfriend and to never stray. Although he doesn't believe that everyone is bisexual, he champions the view that there is the potential in all of us to have sex with both sexes. Will loves the term "sexual fluidity" and applies it to himself. He continues to identify as mostly straight.

SAM

[I] possibly [have a] mild interest in males. At some point,
I may explore that. Presently, no urge to explore. (SAM, AGE 19)

Sam, a 19-year old physical science major, admitted to me that he looked the part of a nerd in high school but now feels he fits in with others in his major. Sam struggled to give direct answers to my questions, modifying many potential answers with caveats. He apologized for "looking a bit burned out," but he'd had a rough night. He did not offer to elaborate.

As a child, Sam shunned large-group dynamics. He preferred to hang out with his best friend, and the two became nearly inseparable. They explored an old factory and played the card game *Magic: The Gathering.* Known as the "weird kid" while growing up and as one of the theater nerds, Sam never considered himself particularly masculine. "Masculinity is a strange concept. I'm not masculine in not being muscular, aggressive, or anything like that. I don't think of myself as masculine or feminine." He didn't play child or adolescent athletic games, in part because his family moved a lot. Although characteristically reticent, Sam found ways to make new friends, nearly always boys, in each new town. Now, in his college dorm, Sam continues to hang out with a few male friends, who are more in line with the druggies than the Dungeons & Dragons enthusiasts.

Sam's first sexual memory was from the fourth grade, when a classmate started puberty early "and someone commented on the size of her breasts." His girl crushes were all secretive and thus not particularly fulfilling. Puberty for him began around age 13. "My voice cracking [was] frequently an issue, types of body hair growing." Sam didn't recall trying to masturbate, though he presumably did around age 13 when the consequences of doing so became a "revelation." It was at that point when he realized, "Okay, I'm definitely getting older. [It was] a division between how I perceived the world and now a new step in my life."

Because his father moved out of the home after his parents' divorce and his mother avoided the topic of sex, Sam did not discover that "new step"—sexuality—from his parents. Health classes became a good substitute for information. In addition, Sam's best friend's mother moved in with another woman, "So I was always comfortable with homosexuality."

Sam began dating his first girlfriend in his junior year of high school, and they started sexual activities, including intercourse, several months later. "She probably initiated because I didn't know what to do or what was okay. I was unwilling to risk doing the wrong thing." They continued to date until several months before our interview, with frequent sex. They ended the relationship because of the distance involved, but they continue to be "friends with benefits" during breaks from college.

Sam has never had a crush on or sexual activities with a guy, although recently he played spin the bottle and made out with both a girl and a boy. "Not meaningful. I see some males as attractive, but [I have] no interest in pursuing them." He's mostly straight because he's "comfortable with my sexuality. [I'm] primarily interested in females and possibly [have a] mild interest in males. At some point, I may explore that. Presently, no urge to explore."

Sam believes "everyone is on the spectrum of bisexuality and people fall on it. I've heard a theory that all females are bisexual and all males are heterosexual or homosexual. I don't give it much credence. Me, I'm attracted to women. I don't know." Homosexuality doesn't threaten Sam. "I'm not afraid of being raped or being disgusted with their sexual practices, so they don't bother me. If they're out, then I congratulate them for their courage."

FELIX

> *People meet me and think I am gay. Yet I'm a*
> *womanizing ass.* (FELIX, AGE 19)

Felix, age 19, tall, thin, fashionably dressed, and quite verbally dexterous, came to the interview with considerable energy. There was an easy nature about him and he was ready to talk, though he visibly began to tire after an hour. Felix's life goal is to market sports products for a large commercial franchise.

In his childhood neighborhood, Felix and his best friend were the "most visible, the leaders" of a small group of boys. Tag, snowball fights, street hockey, and monkey bars occupied their time. "We were the team captains, and we hung out more. He was the cool guy, popular. He could burp the alphabet. I was more academic, and he more into sports. So we complemented each other."

As an early adolescent, Felix drifted between several social groups but was always with his best friend. Together they cut class, smoked pot, drank Russian vodka, and moved cigarettes (to buy the other two). Felix described himself as the "trouble-maker. Always smart who didn't give a shit . . . A mouth and in some fights." He also played the violin. Both are now in college together. In Felix's words, his best friend is "for life. We were never apart."

Felix described himself as masculine with "lots of feminine tendencies such as a preoccupation with appearance, hair, nails, clothes." Yet he swears, drinks, plays sports, and loves women—all masculine traits in his eyes. In college, "every Asian female on campus knows me and my reputation. Five hundred friends on Facebook and I know all of them." He meets women at parties and in the campus women's dorm where he hangs out a lot. Felix is on full scholarship, and he proudly listed the campus clubs he belongs to: Habitat for Humanity, Health Initiative, the *Daily Tiger* (newspaper), Free Clinics, and the Marketing Committee.

His pubic hair sprouted at age 13, the same age he discovered masturbation. He told no one about these two milestones. His "ridiculous" fourth grade health class told him less than he learned from his older brother. His parents later warned him, "We'll kill you if you get a girl pregnant"—their version of a sex talk.

Felix's first sexual memory was a computer generated "snowman getting a boner when he saw a snowwoman." Several early girl crushes would later become girlfriends. In seventh grade Felix was "pretty aggressive with kissing, fondling. I got below the waist once or twice." Real sex, and lots of it, waited until his sophomore year of high school when he had "sex with friends, even though I had a girlfriend at the time." His girlfriend also attended the same Catholic high school, and their relationship lasted nearly four years. Marriage was considered.

Regarding same-sex attractions, Felix has "always been curious and thought of it in my past." In middle school, he had openly gay friends, "and I always feel free with them. I'll call them 'faggot' out of fun." In high school, he helped others "who had sexual identity problems because I was very supportive and I cared." Felix went through a period of wondering if he was "bicurious." When a guy asked him out, "I considered it but more out of comforting him and for him not to be offended. Definitely rumors. Felt I was bisexual because of my haircut, [my] pedicure, [my] care about my appearance. [I'd] talk to girls about their attractions to guys, and I'd add my two cents worth." Because Felix is "a bit femme" even his mother assured him that if he were gay that would be fine. His girlfriend said the same. A college friend shared Felix's same-sex curiosity, and a "girl planned a tryst between us, and so we made out when extremely drunk, but we never talked about it. It didn't bother us. Not disgusted. Shit happens. He was offended when I told others about it. He is straight." Felix will sleep in the same bed as a male friend and physically comfort him.

Felix believes in a gradient of sexuality. Ideally, he'd like to be 100 percent straight. "This is not a judgment, but I believe that experimentation will pass." Now, however, Felix is 95 percent straight, open to anything, especially when intoxicated. Then Felix becomes bicurious. "People meet me and think I am gay. Yet I'm a womanizing ass."

HOLLAND

> *It was an experience. Could not be certain what*
> *I was until I tried it.* (HOLLAND, AGE 19)

Holland, age 19, immediately struck me as someone from another era with his unkempt, long, shaggy hair and clothes from the Recycle, Reuse clothing store. A college junior transfer and uncertain about his future, Holland will likely go into "something medical."

Holland described himself as an introverted child, the kid you'd never notice was around. "I was quiet, teased because of my enunciation of words, socially awkward, dorky." His speech and reading problems contributed to an inferiority complex. His best friend was far more extroverted than Holland, and in middle school Holland became even more "invisible," as he was afraid to talk. Speech therapy cured that problem. In high school, Holland joined a small group of guy friends, and they "hung out and did sports, baseball, touch football, movies, video games, drink, and smoke weed." Eventually, Holland and his friends were known as the stoners and hippies. Holland is comfortable with his low level of masculinity, though with girls he "likes opening doors, paying for stuff." Now he's "socially awkward, so people think I'm closer to them than I am."

Puberty for Holland began around age 11 with pubic hair; six months later he had his first seminal emission while watching "something overtly sexual on TV, can't remember exactly what." The result was confusing because "I wasn't exactly sure what had happened and I didn't tell anyone." Fifth grade sex education and the Internet educated Holland about sexuality, in contrast to his mother's sex talk when he was 15. She told him "not to sleep with dirty girls and to use protection."

Because of his shyness, Holland never told the girls he had crushes on that he liked them. At summer camp when he was 16, a girl put her hands down his pants—his first sexual interactions with anyone and his first "blue balls." This continued for the rest of the summer, but it never went beyond second base. They eventually evolved into a long-distance cybersex relationship, but she objected to him having a girlfriend on campus, and now they're just platonic friends. His first orgasmic sex was in his freshman year in college with an experienced older girl, his first girlfriend. "She asked if I had a condom, and I said yes . . . Condom had issues with, but had awesome time. I was scared that when it broke it leaked." Thereafter, they had intercourse twice a day before she tired of it and reduced it to four times a week.

Holland's first encounter with a guy was with the bisexual boyfriend of a female friend. "We were all drinking, and we made out. Was not sexualized. Whatever, but it didn't do a lot for me.

Was strange but I don't regret it. It was an experience. Could not be certain what I was until I tried it." The uncertainty was because in high school Holland realized there was a spectrum of sexuality and that he "didn't have zero attractions to the same sex." After more life experiences, "I still agree with the above. I'm open minded and more on the straight end of the spectrum. I'm not repulsed by a guy. Generally, I prefer women."

Holland believes he was born straight "until otherwise proven otherwise." Over a year later, on the follow-up questionnaire, Holland remained mostly straight with 10 percent of his sexual attractions, fantasies, and infatuations directed toward guys. He'd had several significant sexual encounters with an ex-girlfriend and a new girlfriend. Holland is comfortable with all sexualities because "I don't see why I should care who people prefer to have sex with." His ideal is to have a relationship with a woman in which both can be sexually intimate with others.

LUKE

> *Girls masturbating don't excite me but it does if a girl gives a huge penis a blow job.* (LUKE, AGE 18)

A recently arrived college freshman, Luke talked quickly, with many questions as he leaned in toward me. It felt as if he wanted to hurry me along so he could continue to talk without interruption. Luke has his heart set on running a casino business.

Luke described his childhood as typical. He was a happy kid with lots of friends. Wanting to be a part of the popular crowd from an early age, Luke played the class clown. He and his best friend had similar interests: "laughter, poker, video, sports team, sports, video." There were "lots of arguments with 'leave my house' and then resolve it two days later." Luke has long struggled to feel that he belongs, so he joined many athletic teams. But he dropped out of high school in his senior year because he was bored and high school seemed useless. He later took the GED test for an equivalency certificate.

Luke described himself as not extremely masculine, although he loves all sports. "I connect very well emotionally with women, and I have many longtime friendships because of this.

Usually I am a very good listener. My passion for learning and closeness is also not very masculine."

Luke was not aware of his puberty until age 14 when his erections became more notable, with the compulsory masturbations. "I felt weird about it, obviously hiding it from my parents. But it felt good, and I looked at pictures on the Internet the first time. I remember that. And I didn't really talk to anyone about that either." Wet dreams have been "very, very rare," but he had one the previous night. In the dream, he followed a girl, and "when I walked to the room she went into, she just attacked me sexually. After I came, I woke up, pretty surprised. I didn't tell anyone, and I'm still actually surprised about it because I've only had one or two of those in my life."

Sex education was covered in seventh grade. "I wouldn't say helpful. Just good score on the test was all I wanted. I trusted my friends more than the class." His mother donated a sex handbook, placing it by his bedside. "I read most of it. No sex talk. Parents were divorced. My dad [lived] in Seattle, and I lived with mom. She asked if I was being safe and if I had any questions."

While visiting his father, 12-year-old Luke felt up his father's friend's daughter "by accident." He liked the feeling of being "naughty and curious." For vacation his mother always took the family to the same place, and one year Luke met a girl there who was "attractive, one year older with large boobs and an impending [imposing] figure, 5 foot, 11 inches." Over the next year they continued over the Internet: "[We] IMed each other about what we would do to each other." Once they were together again for the summer, that's what they did. "I fingered her, and she gave me a blow job." She was the one "who got away." They never saw each other again.

Luke has had three chances with girls he was dating to have intercourse, but to no avail. One had severe emotional issues that he didn't want to take advantage of. With a second girl, in a three-month relationship, there was lots of oral sex, but they were never close enough for intercourse. With his six-month relationship, "she begged me to fuck her, and a couple of times I decided to try it, but then I reached for a condom and lost my erection because [I was] so intimidated by the act."

When I asked Luke if he has had any sexual contact with males, he laughed. "Not gay, never desired." I noted he said he's mostly straight. He explained that he "wanted a male friend to be just like me." Ideally, Luke sees himself as heterosexual and married. Then Luke offered another reason for believing he's mostly straight. When watching porn, Luke is most excited when large penises are shown. "Girls masturbating don't excite me but it does if a girl gives a huge penis a blow job."

Luke appreciates the male body and responds to it accordingly. He easily shows affection to his male friends, and when he's working out he says to them, "Dude, you look really good!" To Luke this is "0 percent homosexuality." He said he'd also feel a little uncomfortable with a gay roommate. "Weird. I couldn't leave the environment. [But wondering] 'Is he looking at me?' would be inherent."

Luke's biggest regret is not having intercourse by now, though he feels this is a "little odd because [I] had so many chances, and [yet I'm] still a virgin. I'm unexperienced." He is, however, very experienced in everything sexual except for that. "I don't want to think or be rushed or nervousness or worry."

MUSINGS

It would be challenging to characterize any of the five young men as typically straight. Will is the only one who has experienced actual genital contact (rubbing) with another male, three times with his middle-school best friend around the onset of puberty. He certainly found it enjoyable, even without an orgasm. His girlfriend encourages Will to explore his gay side, which she apparently perceives as present in Will's makeup.

Holland and Sam each made out with a male in college while drinking or playing a game. Holland felt he had to try it to know for sure that he's straight, and I wonder how many other straight young men feel as though they must test their heterosexuality by making out with a guy. Sam's exploration was during a spin-the-bottle game. Though he has "possibly mild interest in males," which he'll likely explore at some point, he feels no urgent need to go down that road.

Felix and Luke (especially) are curious as to what it would be like to have sex with a guy. Luke focuses on large penises during porn watching, and Felix considers himself to be bicurious, though he has not yet explored his same-sex sexuality or the gayness his mother and girlfriend sense that he has. How typical is it for a straight young man to focus on large penises or to be perceived by those closest to him as having at least some gayness? I don't know, but, again, I doubt that there are many.

All five youths consider sexuality to be a spectrum and do not imagine, despite their heterosexual interests and behaviors, that they are on the extreme end of heterosexuality. This they share with Ryan and Kyle, who are up next.

ryan

So a little while ago, at a party I made out and did some like rubbing and heavy petting with another guy. Just to try it out. (RYAN, AGE 23)

RYAN HAS BEEN AWARE of his slight degree of same-sex sexuality from an early age. As a child he engaged in sex play with two different boys. It has continued through young adulthood with several occasions in which he has had genital contact with a guy. It's all very interesting to Ryan, though his interest in women far exceeds his curiosity about men. As I listened to Ryan's story, I wondered about the degree to which Ryan is turned on by the gender presentation and expression of the person rather than the person's sexual equipment. Pretty men and masculine women both turn him on, but—given his history—he's more attracted to butch women. Infatuation, love, dating, and romantic relationships with guys are out of the question. For him, these belong totally to the province of women.

THE INTERVIEW

A no-show the first time we scheduled the interview, Ryan appropriately apologized for not contacting me to cancel. Even today's date was difficult to arrange as over the past several days we had negotiated several times because of his work schedule. His job, "a temporary service professional," might net him a full-time job, depending on his performance. Aged 23, Ryan wore shorts, a V-neck shirt, and Five Fingers shoes. He brushed his longish dark hair away from his face throughout the interview. Quite animated, Ryan clearly enjoyed talking and responded well to requests for elaboration. Loud laughter, explicit language, lots of hand motions, and perhaps a touch of attention-deficit/hyperactivity disorder characterized his style, and the interview was over in a quick 49 minutes. I'll let him do most of the talking.

CHILDHOOD

Ryan, the youngest of five children, was born five years after his next oldest sibling (Melissa, a lesbian sister). He is the youngest of three boys. His parents were 1960s hippies. "Back in the day, they lived on a commune and didn't touch money." Ryan grew up poor, although now the family considers itself middle class. Their family dynamics were complicated because Ryan was "an accident," one wanted by his mother but not by his father, which subsequently resulted in a rocky relationship between father and son.

Ryan's childhood was dominated by hockey and weight lifting until he tore a muscle in middle school and had to give up both. Next came running and biking, which he continues to love as an adult. His friends were boys with a "few girls interspersed in there." Not surprisingly, Ryan considers himself to be "a pretty masculine dude. I am shaped like a guy. I am very handy. I can do about anything. I helped my dad fix cars, and if something needs doing, I figure out how to do it. If I don't know how to do it already, I will learn how to do it. I can put it together. Like that sort of inner strength I feel like is very masculine." Ryan also has feminine qualities that he cherishes. "I can be very silly and flirty and very bubbly . . . when I want to be. And I am very in touch with my feelings . . . [No] machismo."

Ryan's first sexual memories are from kindergarten and first grade when he did "odd sex play" (a later interpretation) with two boys his age.

> And there was one kid, he was sort of like . . . "Oh, if you don't take your pants off then we're not going to play with my fun toys" sort of thing. And eventually I stopped hanging out with that kid because I was like, "You know what? Screw this! I don't want to do this." And then I started it up with a new kid, and it was more of a mutual thing. It was touching. It was a little bit of oral.

R: Who initiated these interactions?

> In the first one, it was definitely the other kid and then in the second one, I think I started it but then eventually he was primarily initiating it.

R: Why did it end?

> Well, I think for the second one, his parents eventually found out, and they were like, "OMG! This is like crazy shit." And I was like [using a high-pitched child voice], "What, I don't understand? What's going on? We're playing!" And now I understand why they were freaking out a little bit. I think that was about, I want to say, like, a year. It's tough though. It was a very long time ago.

R: How did you feel about these activities?

> Neutral. Just because it was like, "Okay we're playing like this." And the second one, I would definitely say it was in the beginning positive and towards the end I definitely picked up on the fact that his parents wouldn't like this to be happening, if it did come out. Actually, it was funny. His dad was like, "Whatever, they're kids, and they're doing their thing," and the mom was very like, "OMG! NO!" So towards the end I was feeling negative about it because I was worried about the repercussions.

R: Did you have further interactions with them?

Not the first one. The second one, actually in high school I started hanging out with him for a little bit. I don't know his sexual orientation.

R: Did you tell anyone about these activities?

And so, with the first one, when I eventually told my parents I was like, "I don't really want to be doing this anymore, and I am not going to hang out with #1." They told his parents, and they were like, "Oh, he's doing this again? I thought that he had outgrown this." And then for the second one, I think it was towards the second half of it, it was more like common knowledge around the house for both groups of parents.

R: How did you understand the play?

It was like we were like kids playing cops and robbers, but it was like play. It was absolutely play.

R: Do you think it had an impact on you?

Definitely. Also in conjunction with I eventually wanted to go into theater and do theater stuff, and that was really cool because my older sister was into theater and I looked up to her, and my mom was like, "You're getting a little chubby. You're going to play hockey instead." And the hockey kids around here are very like, conservative, and I got a lot of flak for any ounce of any homosexual tendencies for the eight years that I played hockey. That in conjunction with that definitely gave me a little like, I don't know, pause about that sort of stuff.

From these earliest memories, Ryan's same-sex sexuality felt normal and fun for him, but he soon picked up on the fact that it was not considered "cool." A year later, second grader Ryan had his first girl crush—at summer day camp. Here is the backstory: Ryan met a new kid in the neighborhood, Lucas, who was swimming naked at the neighborhood pool. Lucas knew little English, and all the other day camp kids were saying, "'Who the fuck is this kid?' And I was like, 'That's his culture!'" Ryan and Lucas quickly became great friends, and Lucas introduced Ryan to his older sister Linnea, and the crush began. "She was like really nice and stuff, and I really enjoyed spending time with her. She was terribly cute." He never told Linnea about his feelings, and she, Lucas, and their family returned to Sweden.

Ryan's puberty began in eighth grade: "Definitely I got pubes." His memory is precise because it occurred within the context of hockey. "I would go to hockey camps, and you would have older boys who were like, 'I bet your balls haven't even dropped,' and I was like, 'What does that mean?'" Puberty was such a gradual process that Ryan never had the moment when he could say, "Oh, I am a man now." Although he felt late by comparison with other boys, it was a positive milestone because now he had sized up, which made him a better athlete.

His first orgasm was in his uncle's Jacuzzi. "One of the jets felt awesome, and I was like cool! That's fun." Ryan had been masturbating since age 8 with dry orgasms. He told his friends about his experience, and the boys were appropriately awed. His first wet dream came at the age of 14 when he had a fantasy of being at the beach having sex with somebody underwater. "It was some crazy shit."

Porn watching began a year earlier, at age 13. "I always had computer access, and it didn't take me long to figure it out." He could easily hide it from his parents. "I've always been okay with computers, so I would just stash a really large hidden file of porn, and use Kazaa [file sharing software] and all that sort of stuff and download it and put it in a directory that they wouldn't be able to find." Porn has been good for Ryan—an outlet for fun, release of energy, and new things he could learn. Yes, there's "really twisted porn, and you can get a really odd perspective on sex about it. It can definitely skew your understanding of relationships and the way this shit works." For Ryan, however, it was a blessing.

Ryan's source of sex knowledge came from "trial and error," with an assist from his first girlfriend, guy friends, and siblings, especially Melissa. "They were like, 'Oh god! We have to talk to this kid about this stuff.'" Oddly enough, given his parent's openness, they never had a sex talk with their son. His explanation: "My parents were always very overworked. It was just a little bit too awkward for all that, I guess." At one point, it became clear to his mother that he was having sex, and she "hoped" he was having safe sex. He was.

DATING AND SEX

At age 17 Ryan began dating Rihanna, and this first relationship lasted nine months. He broke it off because she was becoming annoying, kind of crazy. "I was like, 'We've been fighting, and I think we should break up.' And she agreed, and that was it." It was good while it lasted, and Ryan learned a lot about sex and relationships. They currently have no contact.

It was with Rihanna that Ryan had his first genital contact with a girl—almost immediately, because they "didn't waste time," and they went all the way to intercourse. "I guess it would have been the second date although we weren't like officially dating. It was more like hanging out." Rihanna initiated it, because she was more sexually experienced, in Ryan's bedroom and unknown to his parents. It was his orgasm, not hers. He shared this amazing experience with friends, who responded, "Good for you!" Sex kept them together until Ryan finally realized Rihanna was "very mothering and naggy . . . I was like, 'I don't need this shit! You're not my mom!' You know, that kind of thing." She was, however, his first love, though now he wonders about it. "Love is complicated because it's just a bunch of hormones passed around, that sort of shit. I felt like I was in love with her."

Ryan's pattern is to have an intense relationship, then remain single for a year or more with random hookups, and then return to another intense relationship. That is, until recently when Ryan had a very serious girlfriend for two years.

> With her, the way you learn to like get to know somebody else's body and when that's happened for me that's been really powerful and has meant a lot. And she was the person I got to know. That sort of learning was definitely the most powerful. I learned a lot about my pattern in relationships and how to conduct myself and my weaknesses as a human being and how to work on myself.

Ryan does not want to marry until he's at least 30. "There's no point." Would he like kids? "I think it would be cool to have kids someday if my life was particularly set up and ready for that, and marriage is a good institution to facilitate the raising of kids. But unless I was going to have kids, I wouldn't want to get married just because [you're] all tied down or whatever." At this point, Ryan believes he's too inexperienced for marriage and maybe there are other ways to "organize relationships, sexual and romantic. And I want to experiment with that and learn more about that sort of stuff." It's not that Ryan is looking to sleep around with just anybody or everybody. Neither is he looking "for the one." Whatever happens, happens, and that is okay with Ryan.

Such a vague "happens, happens" statement led me to push a little further. The one thing that happens all too frequently for Ryan is alcohol.

> I frickin' hate alcohol and sex. It's really annoying because you just want to have sex with somebody and then you're too hammered so you can't have sex with them. It's like, "Dammit, if I wasn't drunk we would be doing it right now, instead of taking you home and throwing up everywhere." It's horrible.
>
> It's interesting because, for most people, they can't get themselves to be uninhibited enough to actually do any of that shit without alcohol and then they can't handle themselves on the alcohol. Even when somebody is like coming on to you and being like, "OMG! I'm so drunk," it's not a turn on.
>
> I would say it's the twist of it. It's made it so I've had more sexual encounters but less sex. It makes it so like people can get to the point where they are willing to actually be all up on someone, but, when it comes down to it, I am very much unwilling to have sex with someone who is hammered and drunk and not able to handle themselves. [Also there's] the whole consent thing. I don't want to do that. It's not what I want . . . I still have this tendency sometimes to just be very on the prowl and being like, "Maybe I can get sex out of you," and being very like, "I will just have sex with everybody," and I end up having sex with nobody. Because you invest in that person a little bit and then they invest in that person a little bit and then nothing gets anywhere.

During his lifetime, Ryan has had casual hookup sex with "fewer than 20" female partners. He rated quite high on measures of sexual curiosity and sensation seeking. Did I mention that he has also had casual sex with four male partners?

SEXUAL AND ROMANTIC STATUS

As is clear from his first sexual memory (sex play with boys) and his young adult interest in casual sex with women, Ryan is a highly sexualized young man, and he is also extraordinarily thoughtful regarding the complexity of his sexuality.

Retrospectively, Ryan noted that during middle school all sexual and romantic attractions were devoted to girls. In senior high, this declined to 95 percent, and after he was in college to 90 percent. However, Ryan makes an important distinction: although 75 percent of his genital contact has been with females, 100 percent of his infatuations and romantic relationships have been devoted to girls/women. One year later, when Ryan participated in our lab study, he reported 85 percent of his sexual attractions and fantasies were with women and, now, nearly all his genital contact. Both years he identified as sexually mostly straight but romantically exclusively straight. In his idealized future, Ryan anticipated that his same-sex sexuality will remain about the same and he might well become a "bisexual-leaning straight" (a Kinsey 2).

Ryan clearly understood himself as being sexually but not romantically fluid. He's never had a romantic crush on a guy.

> I've definitely, like, at a party this last Friday there was a boy that, "Okay, I am just starting to tease out my sexuality towards boys" sort of thing. Just because like again with the early play stuff and that juxtaposed with like hockey where it was years and years of, "Do you like boys? Do you like boys?" And I was like, "What? I'm not answering you." And they were like, "You didn't say 'no,' so I am going to hogtie you and throw you in a trash can!" sort of thing. I am only starting to just like think about that. I have a strong aversive reaction to that right away. It's definitely like hockey years all coming back. The other day, there was a kid,

and if I hadn't had other easier avenues to pursue at the party, I was interested in him. It's an attraction, not a crush.

His first choice is to pursue women, but he'll consider tracking a man. This led to my next question: "Other than the early sex play with those two boys, have you had genital contact with males?" Note here that his answers were more clipped, less elaborated.

No.

R: Did you get close?

Yeah.

R: How did that occur?

So a little while ago, at a party I made out and did some like rubbing and heavy petting with another guy. Just to try it out.

R: How would you rate the experience?

It was positive. But at the time I wasn't interested in taking it any further with that particular person.

R: Was he?

Yes. He is gay. I told him up front that I was just trying it and I wasn't gay.

R: Was it a friend?

No. I just met him.

In terms of women, the "frowzy sorority girl, like tee-hee-hee-hee sort," does not turn him on. Rather, he prefers strong women. "I like somebody that is a little bit more on the masculine side of the feminine scale sort of thing. Someone that can handle themselves."

In terms of men, Ryan is turned on by guys who are "like pretty, not extremely flaming but they are a little bit more on that side of it. They are a little bit more fancy sort of people. Someone more on the feminine side of maleness."

Masculine women and feminine men attract Ryan—perhaps they are not so far apart. Is it the gender presentation that is critical, or is it the genitalia? His response straddled the question: "Both, depending on the person."

Given that mostly heterosexuality is a relatively new concept, even for this millennial generation, I wondered if a mostly straight guy believed in mostly straightness.

> Yeah, [I] definitely believe they exist. I think a lot of the time with mostly straight people in my experience is that they are open to being not straight. And I am open to being not straight. But most of the time, I behave like a straight person.

> R: Is it mostly straight on the sexual side or on the romantic side for you?

> The mostly straight is on the sexual side. On the romantic side, I am pretty much straight. I don't know how to engage in a relationship with a man. I've never tried that before. I am interested, but the right guy has to come at the right time.

> R: Some people believe that mostly straights are just closet cases. Do you believe that?

> No, I don't.

> R: It is clear to you that they are distinct?

> Like, honestly, and in all of the attractions that I've had, I can get pleasure out of both.

> R: Have you met other mostly straight guys?

> No. I don't really talk about it with straight guys because it's the whole, "OMG! We're going to throw you in a trash can."

> R: What is the major distinction between a mostly straight guy and a totally straight guy?

> Probably the biggest distinction is that totally straight people don't know themselves well enough and are a little bit, well, people really like to think of the world as in black and white, and really it's all grey. People like to reduce the model down to one or

zero, and they don't know themselves well enough to, like, actu-ally be able to say it's probably a little bit grey. It might be really, really, really onto the one side of grey, dark grey.

R: What would change this?

Self-understanding and social acceptance. There are a lot of other factors, especially the way that boys are raised that go against us thinking about these sorts of things. Without my sister, the lesbian one, to really help me parse through these things and really think about it and feel acceptance with whatever I do. She's like really weird and totally awesome as well. One of the coolest people I know and would accept me any way that I was. Other-wise, I wouldn't have thought about it. I wouldn't have tried to think about it.

MUSINGS

Ryan is mostly straight, and, though he's personally comfortable with it, he's not certain others would be. He fears some straight guys won't get it and will harass (hogtie) him, and likely neither will the gays. Only his sister Melissa knows. Why hasn't he told his parents? "There is just no need. I guess they would be fine with it, but I just don't talk to them about that stuff." Yet they are "about as liberal as you can get." His mother's nephew is gay ("a special dude"), and the family accepts him and Melissa. Ryan might be sexually fluid because of genetics—same-sex sexuality runs in his family (his sister and cousin)—or because of the hormones that affected his sexual development while he was in the womb—the older brothers and maternal immunity hypothesis, similar to Demetri. Ryan is the youngest of at least three male pregnancies.

Ryan knows he's not exclusively straight, and he doubts that he's bisexual, though he claimed that "I don't even know for myself whether I am bisexual." However, his sexual and ro-mantic interests in women are too present and intense for him to consider himself bisexual. Despite these feelings, they don't replace his sexual curiosity and desire to try out a guy sometime. Ryan is undeniably moving closer to satisfying that curiosity because he recently tried "rubbing and heavy petting with another guy" and it was a positive experience. Mostly straight is where Ryan belongs for the moment, and he likes it—though strictly in the sexual arena. Whether he's on his way toward bisexuality is an open question at this point.

kyle

Maybe I have had thoughts randomly. I think it's just out of curiosity.
I don't think it's something I would ever act on. (KYLE, AGE 18)

A NATIONALLY RANKED WRESTLER when he was in high school, Kyle is honest and forthright about being mostly straight—it's something he never wants to give up because it imparts an edge, an individuality that he treasures. He has no interest in dating guys, but he admits he has felt same-sex desire, which was first expressed when he was 12 with a friend. Although Kyle has predicted he'll follow a traditional heterosexual lifestyle, he does not rule out dallying with a guy. It would not upset him and would reinforce his view that all of us are sexually fluid.

THE INTERVIEW

The day before our interview was scheduled Kyle canceled because he had thrown up, but he wanted to reschedule for the next day. We agreed. Kyle, an 18-year-old freshman, looked a bit haggard and said he shouldn't shake my hand for fear of infecting me, but he managed a great smile. Wearing a T-shirt that announced

"Wrestling," Kyle looked every bit the part: stocky, masculine, and wearing athletic shorts and high top sneakers. He entered college as a premedical student, but after his first semester Kyle switched to a public health policy major. Otherwise, it had been a good first semester for him, and Kyle has formed friendships he believes will last a lifetime. "Here's my second home." Kyle struggled from the outset to form answers to my questions, as if he was trying to find the right words to express what he was thinking or feeling. Whether this was due to his illness, his style, or nervousness about being recorded, I don't know. However, although he was initially hesitant and uncertain, Kyle became increasingly articulate and quite engaged in our conversation.

Overall Kyle appeared totally at ease, especially when he talked about two things important to him: wrestling and being mostly straight. Perhaps no other young man, other than Dillon or Ryan, was as aware or as articulate about the topic of this book.

CHILDHOOD

The youngest of three brothers, with three-year gaps between them, Kyle grew up in a middle-class community in Oklahoma where wrestling ruled. Kyle's entire life has been dominated by sports, and they have garnered him considerable respect and popularity. Just when offers of wrestling scholarships began to fill his family's mailbox, Kyle suffered injuries that ended his career as a wrestler. "It's pretty terrible." Now wrestling and masculinity no longer define him as they had before his injury. "I think wrestling made me not really care how masculine I am. It doesn't matter. I am masculine to a certain extent, but I can also appreciate other feminine things or other masculine or androgynous things."

Kyle's first sexual memory was from age 6. "I found some of my parents' magazines when I was pretty young. I mostly remember this lady on this leopard rug. That's the biggest memory and fantasy I had back then. It was weird but I still got excited by it, but I didn't know what was going on." By second grade his girl crushes began. He never told the girls, of course; Kyle just liked the idea of liking someone. Several of those girls have since become friends, and they enjoy hearing stories about his crushes on them. What appealed to him was how "put together they were, and proper" as well as really smart and good at sports—all things he valued. Kyle told his mother, "Like, 'I have a crush on blah blah blah,' and she was like, 'Oh that's sweet,' or something like that."

ADOLESCENCE

Kyle has never had a wet dream, probably because he began masturbating early, in sixth grade. The first time he did the deed, he was confused about what was happening, and it felt weird. It was a dry orgasm. He knew what to do because a friend told him what to do. Later, his friend showed him when the two boys "did it in front of each other, like once." It was his first orgasm in which something was emitted. The experience was positive because "I was more curious about what other people did and looked like." Kyle told no one. Why not?, I asked.

> I guess just because it was personal and we were pretty young, too. It honestly just never came up, I guess. I just considered it more of a friend thing that we both were experiencing, like puberty, I guess. I didn't really look at it as bad at all. I saw it as, "We shouldn't tell anyone. That would be kind of weird." Obviously. But at the same time, we didn't feel bad about it.

> R: Did you think of it as a gay thing?

> Not really, just like friends. Kind of natural. I don't know.

Porn entered Kyle's life about the same time in sixth grade, when the same friend who showed him how to masturbate also introduced him to Internet porn, which was easy to find ("especially for this generation"). Kyle also learned how to delete his browser history. Porn remains prominent in his life, an easy source of arousal.

Having two older brothers was also a big influence, as were the three *Austin Powers* movies, in teaching Kyle about sex and how the body works. How about his parents? "I never had a legitimate

talk with my parents. It's not like they were trying to hide anything. It wasn't like that. It was just that by the time that it actually came down to it, I don't think there was any point in doing
it. It was just understood that I would find out."

Despite the early influences of masturbation and porn,
Kyle's first dating and first sex came later, during his last two
years in high school.

DATING AND SEX

Kyle hooked up (made out) with many girls in high school, but
his first genital contact was with a friend his junior year, the
morning after a party. At the time they were just friends and not
officially dating. That would come later, in his senior year.

> I felt good about it. She was really, really hot, too. Very positive
> on the chart. I felt like it finally happened. We didn't go all the way.
> We went to second base. Hand job. But it was nice to express
> myself physically and get out. I had always been so conservative.
> It was nice to just kind of get it out.

R: Did you have an orgasm?

> Yeah. I don't think she did . . . I didn't feel like I knew her enough
> to do anything further. I have trust issues, I guess. We didn't un-
> derstand each other enough. We dated too fast. I didn't know her
> well enough before I dated her. You have to fully know someone,
> I guess. People just found out. I didn't tell anyone because I didn't
> want to go around bragging about it. But she told some people.

Kyle had been close to girls before but never "really officially, like, dated, I guess." The girl he'd mentioned became his
first girlfriend, but the two didn't last long because "I had like
commitment issues, I guess." Today they remain friends.

His first intercourse was during "Beach Week" after high
school graduation with another friend. "I don't really regret it,
but I am glad that I waited that long to do it. I actually trusted
the person."

Given these trust/commitment issues, how does Kyle see
his future in terms of sex and romance?

I definitely see myself dating a girl and then marrying her and having kids. Not just because that's the social norm or whatever. It's just how I feel my relationship is going to turn out . . . I want to get married pretty young, so I would say like 25 to 30.

R: Do you want to sleep with as many people as possible or date?

When I got here I realized that nothing really changes that makes me want to have random sex, I guess. I still have urges and things, but it's important for me to have a relationship as well and have that trust and that bond. There are still people I loved back home, and I thought, "Oh, I will go to college and meet someone else." But that hasn't changed so . . .

I might join a frat next semester. That [random sex] might happen a little bit. If it does, I am not going to look at it negatively. It just happens, but I still want to hold strong to my values.

Under the influence of alcohol, Kyle is more likely to "hook up as in make out and things like that . . . Just because I am not a very confident person." This has happened twice. "It loosens me up a little bit like it does for anyone. But whenever something like that has happened, it's not something where I get out of control. It's not like I try to take advantage of drunk girls or anything." Kyle gains confidence hooking up with girls. "It just helps me."

SEXUAL AND ROMANTIC STATUS

Kyle masturbated in front of his sixth-grade male friend and was intrigued by what his friend looked like naked, but he has never had genital contact with a guy. However, he is willing to talk about his mostly straightness. When I ask if he's ever had a boy crush. Kyle equivocates.

Not as much of a crush, and I remember seeing celebrities having, I don't think it was a crush more so than just envying them, which turned into like somewhat of a sexual attraction. But more of just a fantasy. George Clooney. Ben Affleck. That's pretty much it back then. Celebrities are definitely a part. I think it's more of an appreciation . . .

Kyle has also fantasized about female celebrities (Carrie Underwood and Angelina Jolie), but those "were a lot more sexual."

I noted that Kyle selected the "mostly heterosexual" category on his questionnaire, so I asked him to describe what that means to him. Now Kyle becomes more articulate, never stumbling over words.

> For me that just means that I can acknowledge other guys who are attractive. I can rate a guy based on attractiveness, and I can know when a guy is good looking. Maybe I have had thoughts randomly. I think it's just out of curiosity. I don't think it's something I would ever act on. I would say I am mostly straight because I think the stereotype for [a] straight guy is just, you're just into girls, but I think I can appreciate the same sex. I form close bonds with women . . . I can have both a relationship and a sexual relationship. With guys, I would never see myself dating a guy even if it was a celebrity or anything like that.
>
> It's definitely like more emotional. It's more of just like envy. It's mostly celebrities but also adults. People that are the opposite of me, I guess, who are really strong and manly and things like that. It's something that I wish I was but I'm not that much. I guess the envy kind of turns into a little bit of lust. I mean not really. I would never actually do anything.

R: Does it feel repulsive to you?

> No. I think it's something that is natural for some people. I don't think it's anything to be repulsed by. I think it's ignorant. I can see that not being your thing, but it's not something that I would blatantly say is absolutely disgusting. For some people, it is natural. They were born that way.

R: How do you think you got the way you are?

> It took a while, I guess. Growing up, of course, being gay was sort of a taboo. I just think that was part of the world at the time. It's getting less and less like that. That's just how I grew up. My parents aren't extremely strict or anything like that. It was the normal thing. And especially coming to college and realizing that it is

not someone's choice. Even before college, I realized that. Things about gay marriage. That has been a big influence on my views of sexuality just because there are so many good arguments for gay marriage that they just all make sense to me . . . [he makes comparisons to movements for women's rights and rights for African Americans]. My kids are going to be like, "What the hell were you guys doing?"

Kyle has not come out to his family and friends about his sexuality, "which is still bad. I know of other guys who appreciate guys, but I don't think they admit it." His high school friends believe that either you're straight or you're not. Now in college, Kyle sees a shift, and "it's more acceptable for you to say things like that."

I am at the point where I really don't care because it's just who I am, and I wouldn't consider myself gay or anything. I have gotten to the point where I think I am secure enough with myself that I am good to admit it. But there are other guys who definitely have had some degree of interest in the same sex if not acknowledgment of the same sex.

I think that's maybe why the statistics are showing a higher percentage. I think the percentage may have always been that high. It is just that back in the older times no one would ever admit it. You were either one or the other. I think now it's more acceptable for you to say things like that.

Of course, I had to ask about wrestling, with the close physical contact and the potential to respond sexually to the wrestling partner.

Through middle school, I always got a bunch of crap. "Oh you're gay. You wrestle blah blah blah." And honestly, it's probably one of the hardest sports, so those kids had no idea what they were talking about. And then as you get to high school it was viewed as a really good thing because all the really tough kids wrestled. That definitely made me feel good because I was probably the best one on the team. [He lists his achievements.] It got me a lot of respect. I mean you still get the stupid jokes like, "Oh you wear a unitard and you're wrestling guys." But I didn't really care because there was never any thought in my mind of a guy like that when I was wrestling.

R: Do you think there is homoeroticism in wrestling?

I knew one kid who was gay and wrestled. That was a rumor going around in middle school or something. But it's such a tough sport that there is no room for any other sort of feelings besides concentration or whatever and competition. I have never seen wrestling in that way . . . I would say honestly it is less likely. I feel like they would feel awkward probably.

R: How about mostly straight guys?

Just from what I have experienced with the wrestlers, they don't give a shit if someone calls them gay or anything like that. I think that takes a little bit off of the barrier in some respect and they can learn to appreciate other guys. I think there's more mostly straight guys just because they are comfortable enough with who they are and they don't care. I think maybe for other sports it's like that, too. But I think anything who has a very achieved identity would get to the point where they would not care what other people think.

These views were supported by Reuben, a high school and college wrestler who posts vlogs about being gay and an athlete ("Being a Gay Wrestler," https://www.youtube.com/watch?v=zhhndgj6kDY).

Kyle has not been immune from having guys hit on him, which made him feel "really uncomfortable" in high school. "I didn't really like it at all." Yet it was not a totally negative experience.

Once in high school, I heard about this kid and he told this girl that he had dirty thoughts about me or something. It was kind of weird. But I think it would be weird if he told a girl he had dirty thoughts about her. It was just a weird thing. And it kind of made me feel like good. I was like, "Oh, a gay guy likes me." It was kind of funny. In college, I don't think so. No. But it definitely is kind of awkward because that is probably something that I would never act on.

R: How have you dealt with that situation?

I just kind of put it over my shoulder and laugh. It's not like I
get pissed off or anything. I think that's the wrong way to deal
with it. Just be polite about it even though that's not really your
thing.

No one in his family is gay, as far as Kyle knows, though
his next oldest brother is sufficiently secure that he "can appreciate guys so I would say he might be at the same level as me but
a little bit less. He's had a girlfriend for a while. I think it's more
of that acknowledgment." For Kyle, everyone has some degree of
bisexuality, whether they recognize it or not.

MUSINGS

Kyle's level of self-knowledge and self-acceptance was refreshing.
If he eventually marries and has children, he doesn't expect himself to be any less mostly straight. "I still think that I will have
that appreciation for guys, and I kind of like having that. It gives
me a different view on a lot of things. I think that will stay there.
I don't think it will ever be a problem. It's just part of who I am."
In this respect, Kyle recognized same-sex sexual desire, especially
celebrities or adults he envies.

Kyle's sexuality, similar to Demetri and Ryan, fits the pattern that having older brothers can prenatally influence developing a small degree of same-sex sexuality. Kyle is the youngest
of three brothers, and the one just older than him appears to be
mostly straight. Neither Demetri nor Kyle can locate a gay family
member (though Ryan can), which reduces the likelihood that he
is gay by way of genetics.

Throughout his reflections on being mostly straight, Kyle
never expressed romantic desires for males. However, he acknowledged a small degree of lust for guys and made probabi-
listic statements about whether he would engage in sex with a
guy: "probably something that I would never act on." Though
Kyle said he "would never actually do anything," he left the door
slightly ajar, and I have the sense he would not freak out if he

went through it. Given his looks, three more years of college life, and especially living in a fraternity where male-on-male sexual opportunities proliferate and are deemed acceptable as long as they are secretive and with another fraternity brother, I am less certain than Kyle that he'll abstain.

it's about the romance

*He opened my eyes that it is not wrong for a straight
guy to have attractions or crushes on other guys.* (BRADY, AGE 18)

A MOSTLY STRAIGHT YOUNG MAN might truthfully report he
has absolutely no sexual interest in guys, in the same way that
Ryan and Kyle have little to no romantic interest in guys. This
does not mean, however, that he would necessarily reject all such
approaches or is repulsed by them. He would likely divert the
attempted pickup with a "thanks but no thanks" stance. Rather,
he is mostly straight because he experiences or can imagine experiencing an emotional, intimate relationship with another man
that is clearly something more than a typical friendship. He enjoys cuddling with a guy without the pressure of sex and treasures spending countless hours with his "special buddy."

These crush-like infatuations feel normal. Perhaps while he
was growing up he just assumed that other boys felt the same
way he did toward best friends. After all, he always saw guys
hang out together, express positive emotions toward each other,
hug or pat each other, and share intimate thoughts and reactions
with each other. At the time, it wasn't appropriate to define it

as a crush because it seemed natural, and, besides, crushes were what boys had on girls. However, from an outsider's perspective these male-male connections could appear intense. The two boys might be inseparable, cuddle while watching a movie, and even hold hands, depending on the culture. Their relationship resembles a crush. Are they simply best buddies, or is this something else?

These emotional—perhaps we might call them romantic—experiences have motivated some young men to identify as mostly straight. More than once they have fallen in love or become infatuated with a best friend, teammate, or videogame partner, perhaps without mutual reciprocity or even knowing how the other guy felt about it. He might sense a bit of heartache when parting or when his friend moves away or switches best friends. Somewhere along the way he recognizes that something else is going on. In this sense, he is romantically fluid, capable of having crushes on both sexes.

Regardless of what we call these relationships, few mostly straight young men can imagine ever formally or publicly dating a guy or having a romantic relationship with one. This is "too much," like having anal intercourse with a guy, for the sexually oriented mostly straight young man.

For example, while in kindergarten Brady kissed another boy as a dare. It felt normal to have a boy crush, and Brady continued to occasionally have them for other boys throughout childhood and adolescence. Brady interpreted these as friend crushes, not as "real" crushes, which he knew were reserved for girls. "With friends you have, like, a crush but [will] not be romantically involved or have sexual attractions—just a personality attraction."

However, not all boys in Brady's middle school felt the same way about their friendships. As a result, malicious rumors began spreading that Brady must be gay because of these close friendships—and he wasn't dating girls, and he was in the drama club. Once he was in college, Brady talked with his freshman roommate, who turned out to be gay, about what he felt while growing up with same-sex attractions. "He opened my eyes that it is not wrong for a straight guy to have attractions or crushes on other guys." Brady knew he wasn't gay, and bisexual didn't fit him either. "How does one find boys attractive and the polar opposite [girls] also beautiful? I don't feel sexually attracted to males in general. I can tell if they're good-looking but not sexually attractive." Brady now identifies as mostly straight.

Before encountering Jay, a mostly straight romantic, we'll meet Carlos and Kevin, who have distinctive takes on their mostly straight identity. Carlos almost straddles the sexual and romantic in terms of his mostly straight identity.

two romantic young men

I was thinking of [his name] when cuddling with him the other night in his room while watching a movie. (CARLOS, AGE 19)

Carlos thanked me profusely for the interview, which lasted nearly two hours, and said he'd tell others about my work. A 19-year-old English literature major, Carlos grew up in Oakland, California, with bohemian parents who told him early on it'd be fine if he were gay. After all, as a child Carlos painted his nails crimson and dyed his hair purple. His first sexual memory was from preschool when he kissed—"not just a peck but deeply"—a friend, the daughter of lesbian parents. Later, the two families went camping, and the two preschoolers slept "in the same sleeping bag in our underwear, and it was sexually charged with lots of kissing." This was Carlos's "ace in the hole" when he compared the advancement of his sexual activities with those of his friends.

Carlos has never claimed he's a guy's guy. Throughout childhood and adolescence his friends were girls, some of whom became crushes and later girlfriends. Carlos read during recess and displayed mannerisms more typical of girls than boys, which did not endear him to boys. These boys, however, knew better than to call Carlos the "F" word. "In Berkeley you didn't call guys 'fag' because you might fear ten gay guys in high school would cause you harm." Asking Carlos if he would have wanted to be more masculine like other boys in school elicited a barely controlled emotional outburst. "Why would I want to be friends with the rich, white guys who are now in fraternities? You ask if I'd like to be more masculine? You're asking me if I want to be moronic?" Okay, it was time for the next topic.

Each parent had a sex talk with Carlos shortly after he began puberty. Dad told stories about when he was 18 and had his first sex with a girl, their awkward moments trying to have sex, and strategies for how to get a girl in bed. Carlos "didn't know what he was talking about." Mom's version was during breakfast. "I'm groggy and she starts asking me if I have any questions about sex toys, intercourse positions, and if so, just let her know."

The kind of girl who appeals to Carlos is "wild spirited, wickedly intelligent, and generally against almost every social norm one could care to name." He began his dating career in eighth grade with a bisexual girl, with lots of making out. It ended when a member of the crew team called her a *paper bag girl,* which meant that he thought she was "slutty, ugly, had to put a brown paper bag over her head for her to give you a blow job. He said, 'Is that the best you can do?!' " Two weeks later they broke up.

During his junior year, he was dating a girl who was not particularly sexually adventurous. Carlos hooked up with an-other girl while the girlfriend was on vacation. "It was her bed and [included] mutual kissing and making out, clothes removed, and she went down on me. She knew more, so she took the lead. I had an orgasm but not sure if I did anything for her, but I knew I owed her, so next time I made sure. This went on for a week or two."

Carlos described himself as a progressive, pro-sex kind of guy who values the sensitive "new man" approach to male relationships. He finds certain men attractive, but not sexually attractive. One guy in high school was particularly "esthetically gorgeous and now he's an Abercrombie & Fitch model. Very pleasing to look at. I can pick out attractive males as well as attractive females. I've hung out with girls and can say to them, 'Cute guy.'" Wanting to hang out more with guys, Carlos joined the crew team for a male-bonding experience, which was considerably easier to have once he was in college. A particular guy caught his attention.

> I was thinking of [his name] when cuddling with him the other night in his room while watching a movie. Feels very comfortable touching people whether a girl or guy. Would like to experiment with him and see what it's like. It's against my nature to have sexual contact with a guy and am unsure of it and yet curious. I don't ardently desire to be gay/bi. More than half of my friends are not straight, and I miss half the conversation and the words they use. Maybe they have better orgasms and have more of them.

Last week his ex-girlfriend, now at Berkeley, visited Carlos. "I still feel strongly for her. It depleted my condom collection! Long conversation with her afterwards, and we're still in flux." Over the summer after the interview, Carlos bicycled across the country to Portland with a woman, and he now lives with this girlfriend. On his follow-up questionnaire, Carlos continued to label himself as mostly straight, with no sexual contacts with a guy but with guy crushes. He also professed to have keen gaydar: "It is like at home. It's the clothing choices, voice intonation (drawn out syllables at the end of words), accent, elongated vowels, or if he's wearing a rainbow flag." Carlos has plenty of gay friends, most of whom are out. His written advice covered both romantic and sexual relationships:

> Friendships between young men should not be required to lack legitimate emotional content at the risk of being labeled "gay." Such friendships should be socially permitted to involve talking about fear and love and other topics that are normally avoided.

Further, physical contact should not be restricted to the purely masculine, but rather, society should accept hugging and cuddling as valid forms of expressing friendship and comfort. Essentially, I see no reason why such friendships shouldn't incorporate aspects of friendship normally present in close friendships between young women as well as those present in close friendships between young men, and I believe incorporating those things would only make a friendship better.

No one. Period. Should be persecuted and hated for their sexual and romantic preferences (excepting nonconsensual relationships). If two people, or five people . . . love each other and/or want to have sex, that is their business and their right.

KEVIN

> *I wrestled with this guy, my drill partner, and we got very close. We never kissed, but emotionally we kissed.* (KEVIN, AGE 19)

After missing our first appointment because he stayed late after his last class, Kevin was apologetic and rescheduled for later that evening. Despite his manifest masculinity, there was a gentle side to Kevin, most evident in his speaking softly, hesitating before answering, and going off topic. Kevin, a 19-year-old geology major, grew up in a small racially and economically diverse town. Many of his child and adolescent friends were black, poor, and teammates on athletic teams. Kevin claimed he was one of the "nonjackass kids in the secondary popular group," in part because of his humor and his camaraderie with basketball players. He was not great with the girls, and Kevin joined the wrestling, cross-country running, and track teams. He began drinking early, but he wasn't a burnout because he was never a big weed smoker. Kevin always had male best friends, some of whom became "a bit clinging."

His puberty began around 12 with peach fuzz, pubic hair, and, worst of all, acne. Kevin has never been much of a masturbator, at least in the way other guys claim. "I'll look at porn rarely, but most of my [orgasms] are through wet dreams. The fantasies usually involve heavier girls, which I don't think I've told anyone about." These fantasies match his earliest sexual memory, a kindergarten dream: "Me and a fat girl were under-water. I felt euphoric but told no one." Another was "Me feeding a girl. I like big girls. [I'm] attracted to them but don't go after them in my life. It's a fetish but no big deal." Kevin's first instructions regarding sexuality were from his mother when he was in kindergarten. As he grew older, whenever he asked questions about sex, she would refer him back to that birds-and-the-bees story. Fortunately, in his school sex education was every year from fourth to eighth grades.

Kevin describes himself as a romantic because he always becomes attached to girls and develops crushes. For example, in fifth grade he had nine girlfriends; in eighth grade he had his first romantic relationship, which lasted for three months. They kissed, and he touched her breasts and buttocks over her clothing.

Now in college, Kevin wants a girlfriend more than he wants sex. "Never want to touch a vagina or finger one. I'll wait until my marriage night. If I feel the urge, I might, but I don't have that now." Kevin is a virgin: his religious beliefs forbid premarital sex. Besides finding a girlfriend, Kevin plans to join a fraternity to meet guys, and he also plans to lift weights to build his muscles for his currently "pretty manly frame." During the summer after the interview on his follow-up survey, Kevin reported he "very nearly had sex with a girl, but we didn't because my roommates were in the room. Also, I would've regretted it because I didn't like her that much."

Kevin has also never had sex with a guy. "I'm not attracted to phalluses. I don't like phalluses." But he has had many guy crushes.

> I've had crushes on guys. I wrestled with this guy, my drill partner, and we got very close. We never kissed, but emotionally we kissed. This was my junior and senior years of high school. He is a very talented athlete, big dude, first to get an earring. I soon got mine. Badass guy, in a band, singer, songwriter. Girls go crazy for him. He became a good friend right off the bat. I liked most how he talked with me. I'm not closed off to kissing a guy if we had a connection. I've wondered if he was bisexual. We came close to kissing when in private.

Kevin never felt that these feelings indicated that he might be gay, though in fifth grade he thought it would be cool to be gay. He and his best friend were joking around, and Kevin said to a mutual friend, "One thing you don't know, we're gay." It was humor for an effect. In college, he found the term "bicurious" online but didn't feel it exactly fit him. One suitemate asked Kevin during a Truth-or-Truth (no dare) game if he had ever kissed a guy.

> I'm not that averse to kissing guys. Gay guys are like girls in that they won't talk to you if you're not attractive. Hugging a guy is okay. At a fraternity party, I questioned this guy because I think he's gay. He was going after me and touched me. I brushed it off. I didn't like him hitting on me or anything. There are differences in hugs with some "soul hellos," like with my wrestling friend. We'd hug in private, and he touched me in private. [Those] were awkward moments.

I asked Kevin to clarify what he is in terms of his sexuality, but his answer wasn't particularly helpful. "I don't have sexual attraction to vaginas or to sodomy or anything phallic. I have bi tendencies with males, and I think everyone does. I'm bicurious/straight and not closed off to the world." On his survey, he marked *mostly straight.*

Over a year later, on the follow-up questionnaire, Kevin wrote, "Whereas a year ago I was bicurious, I am now steadfast in my heterosexuality." He met a girl over the summer, and they had lunch several times. In his future, he expects to have a wife, and they'll be absolutely monogamous and faithful. Kevin remains a virgin. On his questionnaire, he wrote, "Young men can be very sensitive and tender with friends, without crossing the line of homosexuality. I love my best friends the same way I have loved certain girlfriends."

MUSINGS

Neither Carlos nor Kevin is a typical boy in terms of his gender or sexual expression, and at one time peers perceived both as gay. Carlos rejects traditional masculinity as a deviant way of being whereas Kevin would like to be more masculine, perhaps as a means to be more romantically attractive to guys. Both feel extreme closeness to guys, a bonding that borders on romantic. Each has had opportunities to be sexual with guys and thus to consider whether there might be a sexual component to his feelings. Their conclusions have been similar: "No."

Kevin is clearly more definite about rejecting the idea that his feelings might indicate a sexual attraction to men, perhaps reflecting his general description of himself as a romantic kind of a guy. For his part, bonding with men appears to Carlos to be simply something best buddies do, though he has come closer than Kevin to considering sex with a guy. Each might accept the term *bicurious* to describe himself, although it would be fair to deduce that the curiosity extends toward the romantic rather than the sexual. Kevin's sexuality is difficult to unravel—is his virgin status religiously based, or is he slightly asexual, or is he dependent on his fetish preferences for overweight girls/women (especially feeding them) for stimulation? Carlos and Kevin are sexually straight but romantically fluid. The complexity of sorting through sexual and romantic lives is further illustrated in Jay's developmental history.

jay

I find the penis not to be attractive at all. I don't know why girls like it.
And I also find only men's faces to be extremely attractive. (JAY, AGE 2O)

JAY BRIDGES MULTIPLE RACIAL and ethnic cultures and is thus informed by a number of different interpretations of what should be considered proper sexual and romantic behavior. Are his boy crushes "culturally appropriate" and thus meaningless when it comes to understanding his sexual and romantic self? For now, Jay's focus is on developing a long-term relationship with a girl, not on having lots of casual female sex partners. Yet Jay cannot ignore his romantic attachment—but not sexual attraction—to guys based on their facial features and (especially) hair. Thus he identifies as mostly straight.

THE INTERVIEW

Though he is of Indian heritage, Jay was born in the Middle East before moving to the United States. On several occasions Jay contrasted his unique American experience with his previous life spanning several cultures. Dressed in typical Western attire of blue jeans and a long-sleeve T-shirt, 20-year-old Jay is short, muscular, and plays several sports. He has dark skin, is quite well-spoken, and is an only child. He clearly enjoyed talking about sexual issues, "which is very unusual given my cultural heritage." Jay explained he's had to blend cultures, negotiating between the larger Western culture in which he lives and his family's expectations about appropriate Indian behavior and attitudes. As a result, Jay has become a keen observer of his choices, including sexuality. "I think I would be the same person sexually and invested in women if I were in a different country, but I don't think I would have been with a girl even at this point."

CHILDHOOD

Throughout his life, Jay has played tennis and soccer. They relax him and reduce the anxiety he feels in this "very stressful environment that we are already in. It's terrible." He considers himself masculine in that he's a leader, "good at enunciating what I want to say," and a little bit messy as a person—not in terms of not showering but of "eating like a pig." All his friends had been boys until college, when he was turned off by their sexual competitiveness and chalking up numbers of female sex partners. "I don't get along with people that are of that sort."

Jay's first sexual memory dates to when he was 4 years old. I was informed that I was about to become "the first person in my entire life" Jay has told these details.

> I was worried for my parents to even think of me in that kind of sense . . . I pretended like I had a girlfriend. I was attracted to women at that age, and what I remember [is that] one day we were in the house and we walked over to the—I would have a locket kind of thing I would take from my mom's room. I would walk with her [the imagined girlfriend] over to a table, and I would go under the table with her. She is imaginary, of course. And I would pretend to give her the thing, and it gave me some kind of pleasurable desire.

> R: Was it sexual or romantic?

> I would say sexual because I would pretend to kiss her and things like that.

R: Did you tell someone?

Shameful. Against my culture. Not against my culture, but it's not
looked highly upon.

A year later Jay had his first crush, on a preschool classmate. It was her long, straight hair that today Jay still finds en-
ticing. He was playful with her, and he told his mother but never
the girl. "It was one of those things that I didn't want her to
know. Everyone could know except her."

ADOLESCENCE

For Jay, puberty began around 11 or 12, but again he told no one
what was evolving with his body. He has never had a wet dream,
likely because he began masturbating at the outset of puberty.
How did he know what to do?

I was on a website, obviously. I was watching a girl, and I saw what
she was doing. She was touching her genitals, so I thought I would
touch mine . . . When I saw it [vagina] on the screen, it was the
first time I've ever seen it because people were talking about it at
school. So I went to the website and seeing that actually gave me
a negative [feeling]. I honestly don't know why.

It's hard to describe because it felt good, but I was very scared
as to what happened. I don't know why it happened. I thought I
had done something wrong immediately. It was just not a good
experience.

R: Were you prepared for what would happen?

Not prepared for what was going to happen and not prepared for
what I was going to see. I had never seen a woman's parts like
that ever before.

Fifth grade sex education classes did not adequately pre-
pare him for either the sexual nature of puberty or his energized
sexuality. "How they presented it was, 'Here is a vagina. Here is
a penis. In order for a baby to happen, a penis has to go in a vagina.' And that's it. There's no kind eroticism of it." The focus was
more on "how our bodies are going to be changing, kind of a puberty orientation kind of thing." Yet even this limited information

was useful. "I got a lot out of it. I found that a lot of other kids just laughed the whole time. I was in awe, honestly." Like his first sexual memory and his physical changes, Jay told no one about masturbating or the special websites because he was afraid of what people would say. "My parents still to this day don't know that I do that. Culture again."

Jay has never had a sex talk with his parents, which is common for Indian culture. Indeed, just having sex education in school was an un-Indian thing to experience. When Jay was 18 his father reminded him to practice safe sex. I asked Jay how he thought Indian guys find out what sex is. "I don't know. I really don't know. I think a lot of people there don't have sexual relations until they are married almost."

DATING AND SEX

Jay was 15 when he first had sex, but it wasn't intercourse. He had a best friend, and she became a dating partner because Jay felt obliged to date her after they had sex. "I was also really stupid back then." She initiated it when they were holding each other, and Jay kissed her in a provocative way. She touched him, and from there they went to oral sex. Jay had an orgasm, but she did not. He quickly told his friends, who encouraged him further. He never told his parents. The couple continued to rub "our genitals against each other," but they never progressed to intercourse. Why not? She had the sexual desire and willingness, but Jay was "scared, honestly. I thought I was too young and not experienced enough to know what to do. Not knowledgeable with things like condoms and contraceptives." The two dated for two months.

In his senior year, Jay dated a girl who refused both oral sex and intercourse, limiting their sexual repertoire to hand jobs. After two years of hands, despite her great personality, Jay ended it because "I find physical attraction to be pretty important in a relationship. One of the reasons I broke up with her, sadly." And, moreover, he was not in love with her.

Soon after the breakup, now a college sophomore, Jay had his first intercourse with a friend from one of his classes. "One day she had come over to do homework, and we seemed to get along really well, and I ended up dating her for a little bit. Maybe like two weeks into it we started dating. And a month into our relationship, we had sex." They both agreed they were ready, but for Jay it was just "okay." "I was inexperienced, obviously. I didn't know how to make it feel really good. And, also, I wasn't sure if she was the person for me. I knew she wasn't honestly. I knew that there was absolutely no future."

For the past six months, Jay has been with another woman. Initially, he was not sexually attracted to her, but after they became romantically involved the sexual attraction emerged. They'll likely go their separate ways once Jay graduates. Until he finds his true love, Jay has zero interest in hooking up with girls just for sex, though he thinks that's okay for other guys as long as they don't hurt other people. He's a romantic kind of guy.

SEXUAL AND ROMANTIC STATUS

Jay reminded me that in India and the Middle East, guys hold each other's hand as friends. Hand-holding was, he noted, "absolutely no indication of homosexuality." This was in response to my question of whether he has ever had a crush on a guy—which he has, since the age of 15 ("just good-looking guys"). Jay denied these had a sexual component. Unlike American guys, Jay believes, he's comfortable saying he has boy crushes. "I am very comfortable with my orientation. I am not afraid of judgmental people."

R: What is your distinction between a crush on a guy and a crush on a girl?

Crush on a guy for me would simply be the face area. Just the face when I see a good-looking guy. But a girl involves personality for sure and involves body and everything. And hair!

R: Are there other qualities with guys?

Probably hair also. Hair and eyes.

R: Is there a personality?

No. Just visual.

I then inquire about genital contact with a guy. "No. I am just not attracted to it. My gut reaction is no way. Just no way . . . I find the penis not to be attractive at all. I don't know why girls like it. And I also find only men's faces to be extremely attractive. That's pretty much it."

Gay people elicit no negative judgments from Jay, though he admitted to slight homophobia if a gay guy "is going to lead me on or touch me or something . . . I would get a little physical. I would push the person away. I don't know why. I would push him away." But then, he said, he'd do the same if the person were a girl. No one in his immediate family is gay, though his grand-uncle's daughter is openly lesbian.

MUSINGS

Initially I was puzzled that Jay identifies as both straight (sexually) and mostly straight (romantically), at least until I realized the important distinctions he is making. "I am attracted to guys just face wise. But I am attracted to girls sexually and physically and emotionally and everything. So I would consider myself still as completely heterosexual because I think sexual contact is important." To Jay, if a guy has any desire for sexual contact with a guy, then he is gay or a closeted gay. However, if there is any same-sex emotional attraction (which he has) then he is mostly straight (which he is). Sexuality for Jay is a continuum, not categorical—except when it comes to actual sexual contact, which is likely why he'll never have sexual contact with another male. If he did, then he would, in his mind, turn from straight to gay. There is no fluidity in terms of sexual contact.

Other mostly straight young men possess both sexual and romantic interest in guys, though not always at the same moment or to the same degree. Before turning to our primary protagonists, Joel and Chandler, Ben and Mike briefly share their life histories.

it's about the sex and the romance

BEN

I've had bromances, I guess you could say. And man crushes . . . I would
say I'm 99 percent straight with my 1 percent being those moments
where [I'm] noticing or thinking what would it be like
to have sex with a guy. (BEN, AGE 22)

Ben was born in Korea and soon thereafter was adopted by white
parents from the United States. A senior, aged 22, thin with arm
muscles, black hair, and well dressed in matching shorts and
dress shirt, Ben was easily engaged and readily talked about the
details of his life.

As a child, Ben primarily hung out with his female cousins,
but once he was in middle school it was all guys all the time. His
first sexual memory is a "pretty vivid one" from kindergarten.

> You know the fireman's pole in the playgrounds? I would slide
> down it, and when you slide down it, it rubs against your penis.

I found that, if I were to climb up the pole, then the pressure against my penis would feel awesome. Looking back now, it was essentially just having an extended orgasm without an end for as long as I was holding onto the fireman's pole. So I would climb up it and hold it, onto it for a little while because it felt good and why not?

That was my first experience with masturbation, and it was super young. I would say that's where I realized that I could get sexual pleasure from myself.

R: Did you tell anyone?

I didn't feel guilty, but it just seemed like a private thing. It didn't seem like something anyone needed to know.

Ben next discovered the stair banister in his home, corresponding with the beginning of puberty in sixth grade. It was his first wet orgasm. "I was like, I wonder if it will happen with this, so I climbed up, and I had an orgasm. And it was very strange. It was sticky in my pants, and it was no good. I had to clean up. My parents were out, and I was like, what if my parents catch me cleaning out my pants?" The "banister thing" made Ben realize that "it was just something I could do whenever I wanted to." This turned out to be a more reliable source of orgasms than the slide-show of a bikini festival in the Ukraine that his father caught him watching.

Puberty was a disappointment to Ben. "I wanted to have a beard and stuff like that. I wanted to get tall, grow up big and strong." It didn't happen, but he had many girl crushes, several of whom became girlfriends. One was giving him a blow job when Ben's "puritanical" mother walked in on them. She hurriedly left, and that night his father gave the 17-year-old Ben his first sex talk: "Yeah, you know your mom said she saw you doing stuff with your girlfriend, and we just want to make sure you are being safe." Ben didn't think this was any more helpful than what he'd heard on the third grade playground: "Oh, sex is just being naked and rolling around."

Ben and his girlfriend progressed from oral sex to "real sex," which wasn't so great the first time. Eventually, they "got into the groove of it. Then we started having good sex and switching up positions." The relationship lasted over a year before they began having "like stupid arguments. I wanted to stay together. I couldn't really see straight. I was just sad and desperate. And she was trying to be more realistic because we were going to different colleges."

Ben considers himself highly masculine in the way he approaches girls and his muscles. "I am calculating: What does this girl think about me? Would she talk about me? Also, just in the bedroom, I like being in control of her in bed." With muscles, "I like looking at myself in the mirror, and looking at my muscles gives me a lot of confidence." What kind of woman is he attracted to? One who likes traditional gender roles. "A girl that will let me be a gentleman to her. She's a lady."

R: Are you more of a romantic or a sexual being?

It's weird because those two sides are just constantly battling each other and neither are winning. Except, sometimes, right now the romantic side is winning. But I look back especially like freshman and sophomore year, and there are so many moments where I could have just hooked up with a bunch of girls and I didn't, and that's something that I try to figure out myself. Is it because that sort of fear of not knowing how to approach a girl, or is it health class making me think that if I hook up with a bunch of girls, I will get STDs? Or the fact that I just don't like hooking up with girls with no strings attached? I like the strings attached in a way.

Ben aspires to having a threesome (with two women) before he marries. Now, however, he's in a long-term relationship with a young woman, so the threesome idea is out of the question unless he can convince her to participate.

These stories are strongly heterosexual in scope, so when I asked whether he's ever had a crush on a guy, I was quite surprised.

I've never been with a guy and felt like, "Oh man, I could date this person." I've had bromances, I guess you could say. And man crushes. Sort of like in the fact I just want to like chill and hang out with a guy.

R: Are the bromances different or the same as really good friendships?

I don't know. I feel like even amongst my good friends a lot of them I just don't want to hang out with them because they get on my nerves. Whereas a bromance is always down to hangout and always in tune and wanting to do the same thing. Or I'll come up with an idea, and my best friend will be like, "Totally for sure. Let's go do that."

R: How early in your life do you recall having bromances?

Definitely kindergarten.

Has he ever had genital contact with a guy? It's Ben's ambivalent and at times contradictory responses that are critical here.

Because the idea is kind of disgusting to me. I've wondered, "Hmm, what would it be like to hold a penis or to have anal sex with another guy?" The thought has crossed my mind. And I've also thought, "Well, I masturbate so much I would give awesome hand jobs." But actually doing it, it's not something I would really want to pursue.

R: What part of you isn't 100 percent straight?

I would say I'm 99 percent straight with my 1 percent being those moments where [I'm] noticing or thinking what would it be like to have sex with a guy. That's actually when I'm watching porn and its almost sort of narcissistic jealously. When I see the guys in porn that are really jacked, really muscular, and are just going to town on the girls in porn. Sometimes I notice myself noticing his muscles and his body and the way that he moves and what he is doing on the screen. Almost like a narcissistic identification with him.

R: If a guy came onto you, what would you do?

Actually, it's happened. Some of my gay friends and I just totally play it up. I'll act gay and slap his ass and shit. Because it is uncomfortable for me, turning it into a joke makes it into I own it.

I own the fear. It shows to other people that I am not afraid. If one of my gay friends was coming onto me and I was just like squirming, I would feel more vulnerable. I guess it has happened, not intensely, but I have been hit on by a gay guy in a club a little bit, and I just kind of played the ignorant card. He was being super nice and complimenting my clothes, and I was like, "Thanks man! I got this at American Eagle."

Being mostly straight for Ben is a complex matter that includes both romantic and sexual desires. He's had bromances (boy crushes) from a very early age, and some have been intense. He's wondered what it would be like to have another's penis in his hand, and he's admired the bodies of male porn actors. Given these feelings, Ben knows that he cannot claim to be exclusively straight—so he has chosen to identify as mostly straight.

MIKE

Being bisexual wouldn't be so bad. [I'm] not uncomfortable with it . . . [I'm] open to the possibility of pursuing men because [you] never know who one can fall in love with and [it] could be a male. (MIKE, AGE 21)

Mike, 21 and somewhat overweight, grew up on a small Midwestern farm and is currently majoring in the humanities. Mike believes that he's not overly masculine because he doesn't like sports and doesn't have strong male friendships. But he is not without masculine traits because, as he pointed out, "I don't really worry too much about appearances, about politeness. I stay calm and levelheaded and control my emotions. I like to be crude, and I like to get dirty." Mike sees himself as an outsider because he believes that "rules don't apply to me, regardless of what others think. I rebel against hard and fast rules, both negative and positive."

Mike's childhood was dominated by two male friends. Together they were the Three Musketeers. They were constantly together creating tree fortresses, having sword fights, and building grand fantasies of stealing guns to fight the FBI and of living together forever as an alien race. He was particularly close with one of the two, and their relationship was intense. Mike thought they would be best friends for life, though it hasn't worked out that way. They imagined that they would grow up and marry each other, and that, too, hasn't worked out.

Mike's first sexual memory was pretending, when he was 5, that his blanket was a girl and humping it. He was excited by the notion that his parents might catch him in the act. (They didn't.) Wet dreams of having sex with random women on the street were frequent, until he learned how to masturbate at age 15. "I had an erection and felt compelled to play with myself." His fantasies were again of random women. Sex education was succinctly presented in a sixth grade seminar in a hospital setting to escape the highly controversial political implications of being "school-sponsored." Before that, Mike didn't know vaginas existed. "I thought girls had a butt that went all the way around, and I put the penis in there, and that's how babies were made." His parents didn't talk to him about sex until his late teenage years when they instructed him, "Don't do anything stupid." That kind of sex education wasn't particularly helpful.

Mike's first genital contact with anyone occurred in his freshman year of college after an environmental club meeting. The two went to a park, ordered takeout pepperoni pizza, and made out. Then unexpectedly, just as he thought they were finishing, she lifted her skirt. "I felt her breasts and played with her." She told him she had lost her virginity in eighth grade. Mike was hugely relieved that even though he was inexperienced, he could figure it out when the time came. He gained the confidence he thought would be helpful—it wasn't—several weeks later when they tried intercourse in Mike's room. There were major problems: "I'm not circumcised, and it didn't work because the foreskin didn't come down. Tried it and she ended it. Over beers she said no longer would we do these kind of things."

Sophomore year of college Mike established a six-month relationship with a woman he met in the dorm. Everything went better, but not great.

> Was the first functional relationship I had. Never said we loved each other, weird. Left me with a lot of baggage. I was warmer and she colder, and then she cut it off. Was [it] the sex life which

was not satisfactory? She was a virgin and wanted to lose it. She has a low sex drive, and it was painful for her. We tried four or five times, and I did have an orgasm several times.

The baggage was I kept trying harder to get her attention and pressuring for more sex and felt like I was inadequate and not doing things right, not trusting people and opening up.

True love would wait until his current relationship.

In between these two events, during his freshman year of college Mike had a "gay experience" with a male friend in the same dorm. Again, notice the ambivalence.

I didn't know he was gay, and we went to a party and hung out. Kissing and made out. We dropped acid the next day, and I freaked out. Felt weird and not sure I enjoyed it. He was trying to have a relationship with me, and I was giving him half-ass replies.

R: What did you guys do?

Kissing, open mouth with tongue.

R: Why did this occur?

Complicated question. I can't see myself identifying as gay, and maybe that is cultural baggage. It wouldn't mesh with my personality. Physical contact made me feel submissive and me smaller and him bigger on top of me. Couldn't see myself doing the kissing. Not pining over it, and I did not throw up like [when I eat] food I don't like that much.

I asked Mike to trace his developmental history of sexual and romantic feelings, especially during childhood and adolescence. As a child, he had many girl crushes and several "mild, maybe sexual crushes on a guy." One guy was on the baseball team "who was very pretty. Male crushes that were not sexual but still crushes, strong attachments to guys." This pattern continued through junior high, including the desire "to experiment and see if I like it [male sexual contact] more than I think I do. I'd worry about the judgment of others." In senior high school Mike was friends with several gay guys, and given that many of the girls he knew were "experimenting with other girls and bisexuality and being in theater, I heard rumors that my old friend had gotten a blow job from a gay stranger. I had had an infatuation with him [friend], but I also had a strong crush on this girl."

R: And now?

Occasional sexually attracted to males, not strong, and more platonic crushes on guys . . . Sexual attractions to guys confuse me, and I'm not sure I'm interested in them. In an ideal world, I'd be okay and indulgent with that part of my sexuality. Don't feel comfortable emotionally with it or with experimenting because once I do it then I open myself to other things. I don't think I could handle that.

Being bisexual wouldn't be so bad. Not uncomfortable with it. If I could be like Walt Whitman was with his some of his friends. I could stay masculine and open to the possibility of pursuing men because [you] never know who one can fall in love with and [it] could be a male. Feel uncomfortable with gay culture and subculture.

Comfortable with hugging. Can be awkward. Fear how it is interpreted and how they will react . . . It is strange territory because of our culture . . . I read Judith Butler [a feminist, queer philosopher], and I believe it. Makes sense to me . . . [that I'm] 10 percent to 15 percent attracted to men and other to women, and all express it in different ways.

Not surprising given his reading of Judith Butler, Mike believes his sexuality is a learned behavior and thus he is sexually and romantically fluid. He was confused when he asked his childhood friend to marry him and the response was laughter. This was the "cultural cue" that turned Mike away from a life of same-sex sexuality to heterosexuality. According to Mike's reckoning, his mostly heterosexuality is the residue.

MUSINGS

Ben and Mike have struggled making sense of their fluid sexual and romantic feelings. Because they both experience sexual and romantic attractions to both sexes, they're not quite sure where they belong on the spectrum. Neither denied his history of rather explicit sexual and romantic feelings toward guys, though both were clear in having considerably stronger heterosexual than same-sex sexual and romantic attractions.

Perhaps both young men are between Kinsey 1 and 2 points on a sexual and romantic continuum, with Mike especially coming close to the border of a Kinsey 2. Each bases his sexual and romantic identification on the combined strength of these feelings and compares them with his feelings toward women. The net effect is that both determine that they are mostly straight. Joel and Chandler also faced these dilemmas.

joel

I think there's so many pretty girls around that I don't need to really be attracted to this guy. I think it's out of my way to have a sexual relationship with a guy. I wouldn't object to it if frustration arose and there was nothing better to do. (JOEL, AGE 23)

AS A YOUNG CHILD, Joel played sexually motivated games with other boys, unaware that adults might be alarmed by such behavior. Joel believed that these amusing activities were common among boys and would have no impact on his future sexual behavior and identity. Since then, more opportunities to display or act on his homoeroticism have presented themselves, including his willingness to give a blow job or participate in threesomes in which another guy is present. In addition, Joel has a history of boy crushes and becoming "touchy-feely" with male friends. Perhaps of all the mostly straight guys I interviewed, Joel had the most explicit congruence of homoerotic sexual *and* romantic experiences with guys—genital contact and boy crushes. These encounters do not cause Joel to question his straightness. Rather, they are simply part of the fabric of his fluid life.

Joel, 23 and of mixed ethnicity and nationality, arrived after changing the interview date several times. He was graduating from college and was behind schedule in preparing for his large extended family's arrival for the ceremonies. This included, he dejectedly announced, shaving his month-long beard. An only child born to aging parents who tried for nearly twenty years to have a child, Joel dressed in total black and chewed what appeared to be tobacco snuff during the first few minutes of the interview. There was a softness and low-keyed sincerity about him. An anthropology major, Joel spoke slowly and deliberately, and I wondered if there might be a language issue, as English was his second language. Yet his spoken English was perfect. Tall and lanky with light skin, long, dark hair, and considerable eye contact, Joel's college nickname is "Euro Macho." After being initially anxious, which might best explain the changes in interview times, Joel "grew into the interview," such that by the end he asked that I keep in touch with him.

CHILDHOOD

As a child, Joel played nonstop soccer and tennis, like his friends. Joel believed as a child he never measured up to the American ideals of masculinity. However, Joel takes great pride in always expressing his views. Indeed, Joel didn't keep his thoughts to himself, though he claimed not to broadcast his strong opinions in an obnoxious way:

> I usually let things run their course and let people finally accept that I was right. Kind of in that way I'm not very bitchy. I don't freak out and start stressing out about things. In that way, I would say I am masculine. I won't change my opinions easily. I won't express them easily either. Other than that, I think I am very experimental. I will try new things in any situation.

At several points in the interview Joel warned me that it might appear that he's contradicting himself, but he isn't.

Joel said he also has a feminine side that includes—his words not mine—being moody, giving up easily on short-term tasks, being easily influenced in conversations and switching too easily, being too adaptable, and speaking the language of whomever he's speaking with. At the very least, Joel's characterization of femininity was not positive. I saw the contradictions between his stated masculine and feminine selves, and there would be more.

Joel's first sexual memory was just before he was circumcised at age 6. His family lived in an apartment complex, and the gardener had a 4-year-old son, also uncircumcised. The two boys often played together, and, being the last to be circumcised in their group of friends, they were quite anxious about its inevitable due date.

> Most of my age group had it immediately when they were born, and before it always used to be 6 or 7. There was a big celebration and traditional sort of doctor characters who weren't really doctors but they were specialized circumcisers. So we had this anxiety. We used to combat it, so we would come up with this game where we would play as if someone was a circumciser and the other one was a patient and we would switch back and forth, and it entailed maybe touching the penis a little with stuff.

> R: Did you tell anyone about the game?

> No. I kind of knew it was a little weird. Why would I tell my parents? I didn't really tell them what games I played like soccer or whatever. I didn't exactly tell them what I did every day.

> R: Did this memory have meaning for you?

> I think so. Every once in a while I will think about it and say, "Ah, that was brave of us to do." I guess I initiated it. He was younger than I was. He was playing along and not seeing anything wrong with it. For us, it was kind of fun and exciting. I never thought it was a horrible thing that we did this game, like we were perverted kids.

A girl from his tennis team was Joel's first crush when he was 8. She was playful, lanky, fast, and very active—all characteristics of girls that remain appealing to Joel today. The crush was mutual, and all their friends and families knew, but nothing came of it.

ADOLESCENCE

A late-maturing boy, Joel clearly remembered his first orgasm. Yet, before that, during middle school, Joel said he had sex dreams with dry orgasms. "I don't know if it could be classified as an orgasm [because there was no emission]. Definitely something along those lines." His first wet orgasm was through masturbation, around age 15, after he went to soccer camp.

> My school had a soccer team. It was a pretty good soccer team. It was a bunch of rich people who could afford it, and I was sort of tagging along. We had older guys and younger guys, and we just spent all of our time together. We were in the mountains, and there was nothing to do. We would do soccer during the day, and it wasn't a mountain resort or thing like that. It was a hotel where you just eat and then you are sitting around. At that point, there was an older group of kids who were teasing me about masturbation. Trying to teach me or whatever. I learned about it for the first time. They kind of went on for a while, and on the soccer trips everyone was talking about masturbation because it was so new and exciting. So my friends would kind of show off.
>
> We had a communal masturbation setting at night. They would ejaculate and make fun of the people who couldn't. I don't think I ejaculated then but sometime during that year. I was just experimenting and trying it out.

Joel wasn't sure how he learned about sex and his developing body, but my question about having a sex talk with his parents elicited a strong negative. Though his mother was a "progressive lady," there was never a sex talk, and he had to rely in part on observational learning. Because both parents worked, leaving Joel home alone, when they were home Joel recalled times when he so much wanted to be with them that he'd run into their room while they were having sex. "They kind of laughed it off and said to go away." The basic knowledge was covered in the school's curriculum. "It was kind of a requirement that no one wanted to do . . . I remember [that the teacher] went on about sex and morality. No one could figure out what she was saying."

More influential was porn, beginning on New Year's Eve when Joel was 11. While his parents were drinking and dancing on the tables with friends, the kids stayed home and watched the sex channel all night. Joel believes that perhaps he now watches too much porn because, "Well, if the Indians are right and there are certain number of ejaculations you can have before you die like heartbeats, then it's probably bad because it's not necessary in that way. I think nowadays I would rather it didn't play a role, but it still does. I think in general it is a little negative." He doesn't have a need for porn because for the past eight years he's always had a girlfriend. "Not since I was like 16 I have had needed it as a tool to pass time or to crunch my sexual appetite."

DATING AND SEX

In terms of girlfriends, Joel's first serious relationship began in his sophomore year of high school and lasted off and on for five years, eventually ending when he was in college. It was also his first genital contact with a girl. He was the more sexually experienced because he "thought about it more. I masturbated. I don't think she ever masturbated." Two months after beginning to date, Joel initiated sexual contact.

R: How far did you guys go the first time?

Just touching. I was touching her, and she was touching me a little. Mainly me touching her. No orgasms . . . I really liked her. I had had chances before, but I didn't take them. I thought it was a good time to do it.

R: Did you tell anyone about it?

No. She was my closest friend, and it was kind of a dramatic relationship.

R: Did you two have intercourse?

We started trying, and I guess it was really difficult for her, unusually [so]. For the next few years, on and off, we tried, but it never actually happened although we wanted it to . . . It slowly got better, but I never actually could. I think it's because it was very easy for me to complain when she was with me. The funny thing is, after I came here, the next week she lost her virginity to some other guy. She said I couldn't complain to him because I didn't know him . . . Maybe he was more persistent.

R: Who initiated the sexual encounters?

It was very nice because, at that time, she was a boarding student, so her family was elsewhere in the city. They had no clue, so she could get out of the dorm whenever she wanted. And my mom had to share their office right close to school, and I had the keys for that place. So we would just go there, and it was office building where the whole floor was to herself. That was nice. We just did a couple hours of foreplay. Really long extended periods of foreplay and then we would sort of try it, and if it didn't work, like a hand job or something.

It was kind of like three years of trying. It was very good at the beginning, but it progressively got worse and worse, and by the last year of high school it wasn't very positive anymore.

She was his first love, and now he is in love with the woman he has been dating for over a year. Joel sees himself married. "I don't want to be too old and not be married. I don't want to be 40 and not be married." Until then, Joel would like to have more sex partners, without making it public, without seeming to be "'that way.' It's not my goal. I would like to potentially, but I in general prefer to be in a romantic relationship and see how that evolves . . . I don't want to sleep with 50 people. I want to sleep with one person 50 times."

During sex with girls is when Joel becomes "most feminine. It's fun to act like 'the other.' Change roles. Not change roles. Yeah, I can see myself changing roles in bed with a girl more easily than sleeping with a guy. I don't do it too often. But if she wanted, I would be down to do it if my girlfriend wanted to do it more . . . After a few drinks, you don't know what's going to happen."

Joel's biggest regret was not having sex with a really cute girl who'd had a huge crush on him. He could have done it with her but didn't. "I am kind of proud of myself. I was kind of loyal to my high school girlfriend, and I didn't want to. I was more [a] prude in the situation . . . I still regret it." Then Joel recalled a girl he shouldn't have slept with but did, "and then said good-bye. But she was asking for it."

SEXUAL AND ROMANTIC STATUS

Joel had early circumcision sex play with a boy, a communal masturbation session with the boys' soccer team, and stated that changing roles during sex with a woman would be "easier" than sleeping with a guy. Do these references have meaning for Joel's current sexual life?

In terms of his postpubertal self, Joel's first genital contact with a guy was during his freshman year of college. A fellow student who lived down the hall initiated the interaction.

> He's gay, and he really wanted me to be gay also. So he said, "Oh, I'm going to test you," so he put his hand down my pants and was trying to arouse me, but I wasn't feeling antagonistic against him. I was not aroused either. Just to prove him wrong, I didn't get aroused.

R: How would you rate that experience?

> Kind of sarcastically positive. It's positive. It wasn't like, "Oh, I'm so happy about it." Something to laugh at now.

R: How do you understand your sexuality in this regard?

> I think there's so many pretty girls around that I don't need to really be attracted to this guy. I think it's out of my way to have a sexual relationship with a guy. I wouldn't object to it if frustration arose and there was nothing better to do, but at that time I was still in love with this girl . . . So it did not happen anyway. But as I said, it's kind of out of my way and an extra of effort on your part.
>
> I never get aroused by looking at a guy walking down the street, although I do get aroused by girls walking down the street. I watch them. I would never watch gay porn either. I don't think it's arousing. So you're a man. I'm a man. What is there to be ashamed of? It wouldn't be like you have such nice curves or you have such a nice body. I don't know. It's not about finding

someone sexy, it's more about like a battle of wills . . . It's kind of like a peeing competition. Guys will get in a row and try to see who will pee the furthest. And then you would never say, "I can see your dick." It's like a competition and a competence situation. I can't really phrase it too well.

R: Have you ever had an orgasm with another guy?

No. Never highly motivated to seek it.

R: Do guys often come onto you?

It hasn't happened in a year maybe . . . The last time it happened was when it went the furthest. I really like oral sex. I would have given him a blow job, [but] he couldn't get an erection. I wouldn't have minded doing it.

He posed as highly masculine, but it turns out he is gay. He also had a girlfriend he was going to marry. They were engaged or something.

In terms of his romantic self, it's not unusual for Joel to become physically, emotionally, and intellectually in tune with his "really close friends, or they become really close friends." He identified two guy crushes. "The earliest was my freshman year here. But he's my best friend. I have a crush on him. I will give him a massage. We are very touchy-feely with another . . . Actually, I had one more. But that guy died. That was very sad."

It is noteworthy that on his mother's side Joel has a lesbian cousin and both he and his parents are progressive when it comes to gay rights, unique among their ethnic groups. But I have one final question for Joel: How is he different from a straight guy? According to Joel, straight guys look and move in a "boring way. There's a lot to explore in movements. I like to dance. There's a whole range of movements that you can express."

MUSINGS

Joel described himself as mostly straight largely because he admires the beauty of the male body, especially its expressiveness. He's had opportunities to see the male body, on several occasions in college, including several threesomes involving a girl and another guy. Joel wasn't highly motivated to orient himself toward guys in these situations, though he was willing to give a blow job.

Also telling are the intense male crushes he's had throughout his life and his strong preference for masculine guys who do sports and "aren't afraid to use their body and get active and brave the elements." With these guys Joel loves to cuddle and be intellectually engaged. Though Joel has both same-sex sexual and romantic inclinations, it's difficult to imagine Joel dating a guy or having anal intercourse with a guy. Without doubt, however, Joel identifies as mostly straight.

chandler

*Mainly because if I was kind of alone with this guy that I was attracted
to and there was no possible way that the outside world could know
about it, I probably would do it.* (CHANDLER, AGE 18)

IF I WERE BETTING, Chandler would be one of the young men
most likely to transition from mostly straight toward something
more traditionally bisexual. He says he's in the closet, but it's
never quite clear what he's in the closet about. His sexual and
romantic orientations toward women are clear and highly trea-
sured. The same cannot be said about his orientation toward
men. Chandler has never made genital contact with another man,
though he's "attracted to male genitalia" and "willing to experiment." He's had opportunities, but has not yet said yes to them.
In terms of romantic involvement, there's a guy who lives in his
dorm who enchants Chandler. In his next three years at college
these issues will likely be resolved.

THE INTERVIEW

Chandler, an 18-year-old freshman, immediately gave me fair
warning, with an accompanying sad look, that his answers might

be influenced by the fact that his long-term relationship with a young woman had just ended. Slight in build and height although he works out to develop his masculine appearance, Chandler has dark hair and a great smile, and he wore blue jeans with a long-sleeve, stylish sweater to the interview. He immediately became engaged in the interview, which became less a conversation than a Q & A session. Chandler leaned forward eagerly in the swivel chair waiting each question, then swirled away from me to quickly answer the question, then swirled around to face me and lean in for the next question. Though Chandler whispered that few others know about the complexity of his sexual and romantic attractions, he was strikingly open during the interview about these issues—with clearheaded insight and reflections. If this was him sad, I could not tell.

CHILDHOOD

Chandler's best childhood friends were initially girls, but he turned decidedly toward boys in middle school. Chandler participated in karate, swimming, and tennis, and then added rowing in high school. He considers himself "pretty up there" in masculinity. "I think that's a large reason why I am unwilling to step out of the closet, because I think a large portion of that will be lost." Chandler also views himself as feminine. "There's a stereotype of guys that they don't really like to talk about their feelings. I definitely feel like I kind of need to, otherwise I'll go crazy. I just like sitting down and discussing what I feel with people. It's just nice. On the flip side, I feel like I do sports. I work out regularly. I like to stay fit."

His first crush was on a girl Chandler "got kind of crazy over" after the two became good friends. As you read this, remember they are fourth graders.

> That whole notion of liking was very prevalent at that time. We kind of told each other and got very embarrassed. She was very smart and very talented. That was definitely a big plus. I felt that we had a lot of things in common in the sense [of] our attitude towards school and life. It was very much like, enjoy what you can, but at the end of the day you go to school to learn. That really

appealed to me about her. She went out of the way to challenge herself, and that also appealed to me. Sexually, I don't think there was anything there. I think it was just an innocent crush.

Chandler told several of his best friends about the crush, which turned out to be a light-hearted conversation. There was no drama, and the two never dated.

ADOLESCENCE

Chandler's first sexual memory was of an incident with a girl as he was on the edge of puberty. Her interest in his visible erection piqued his own interest in his erection, which eventually motivated his first masturbation.

> We were watching these YouTube videos, and there was this one really attractive woman in a video. We were like 11 years old. I am pretty sure I had an erection at that point. She was very curious as to what that was, and then I remember we were kind of unsure, and I kind of nudged at it a little bit and it felt good, and we didn't really act on it or anything. That's the first time I remembered something like that.

R: Did you understand at that time what was going on?

> I did not. I had some friends that were older than me at the time, and I kind of asked them what all this was about. This is when I found out about sex and reproductive organs and all of that. And that's also when I found out about masturbation. Eleven or 12 was when I started doing my thing. So, yeah.
>
> At the time, it was kind of just like a new experience. I wasn't feeling overwhelmingly negative towards it or anything. I had no idea what the hell I was doing . . . I remember after she left, I came back and watched the video again, and I was aroused again, and I started messing with it and it felt good . . . I started rubbing my crotch area and it felt good, so I just kept kind of rubbing it. I didn't do the standard wanking motion or whatever. I just kind of started rubbing it and it felt good. Only in middle school when people started making these crude gestures I figured maybe that is what you should do. So for me it was more like that.

R: Did you tell anyone?

No, I didn't tell anybody. I knew I couldn't talk to my parents about it because of that kind of upbringing, and I felt like it was too early to talk about it with my friends . . .

I remember a lot of times afterwards when I would come I would often feel really guilty or really bad about it. But the first one I remember I was like, "Oh, it felt good." In sixth grade, I kind of felt guilty because of the stigma that was attached to it, and I was like, "What am I doing?" It was more like at that time I could be studying or I could be working but instead I am doing this.

R: Do you think it had an impact on your life?

I feel like it did in the way I didn't really intend it to. Right now, I feel like I am kind of open with all this and I really want to celebrate sexuality. I am that sort of person. And I felt that if I had maybe told my friends about that incident then maybe I would have been embarrassed and I would have tried to hide it and stuff.

Although one of his friends talked about masturbation and other taboo stuff, in general Chandler and his friends were all "in the same boat and were hiding it or not telling."

By age 12 Chandler was masturbating on a regular basis, with an assist from porn. Later he had wet dreams (images of an older girl). Twelve was also when puberty began, defined by Chandler as "feeling sexual attraction to girls." He liked puberty, especially his voice deepening.

R: Was porn positive or negative for you?

Definitely in the beginning it was very negative. I felt really guilty for even watching these videos. But I guess that all changed when the stigma towards it sort of flipped. I remember, at least in the beginning, I would always watch soft core, and I would feel really guilty if I didn't.

If my stigma didn't change in my seventh grade class it probably would have been terrible because in seventh grade there was a huge reversal in my head and it suddenly became okay to watch porn. It was completely natural, and now it is completely natural.

R: Did you feel you were watching too much porn?

Definitely in high school. Probably in ninth or tenth grade I spent a lot of time watching porn and masturbating. That all changed after I started trying out this committed relationship thing.

Chandler's sex education came from the neighborhood kids and from a "really thorough explanation" in fifth grade sex education class. This was in the absence of any conversation with his parents about these matters, though his father had to sign the Family Life consent form for the school class. Sex is a taboo topic in Chandler's home. "When you mention the word 'sex' or anything remotely related or condoms or safe sex or STDs, there is this giant panic button and it comes into everybody's eyes . . . It's really silly."

DATING AND SEX

In seventh grade English class Chandler asked one of his friends out. "Yeah, sure," she said. Early dating meant holding hands until one day Chandler kissed her, which was "great." In eighth grade, they reignited their passion with genital contact. "I fingered her. She definitely didn't orgasm or anything, but I just remember my hands were getting really wet and I was really into it, and she kind of grabbed at my crotch a little bit, but I didn't take it out or anything." That was as far as it got because time alone was difficult to arrange. Several other girls followed, including one experienced in the ways of sex. They went "pretty far" but no genital contact, though they came close.

After his recent one-year relationship ended, the one that devastated him, Chandler has been "kind of leaning towards the sexual side of the scale. I can't see myself in a relationship for a long time. It's just so emotionally investing." That said, Chandler will never forget the "absolutely amazing" relationship that had just ended. "It was phenomenal . . . It's nice to have some sort of security net." The problem is Chandler doesn't want a monogamous relationship. "Ideally, no. Because a large part of why this ended was that I felt a little bit too constricted sexually." They were quite sexually active (especially while watching the *Lord of the Rings* movies) and faithful. Although Chandler went to various parties without her, he didn't bring girls home.

Chandler's first sexual intercourse was not, however, with the girlfriend but was earlier, with a friend after consuming alcohol together. Chandler took this opportunity to educate me about a common fact regarding how his generation woos sexual partners (leading up to intercourse).

> There was a lot of sexting going on with me and this other girl. That dynamic is totally different than even like hooking up. There's a lot more trust in that than you would expect. When you hear the term sexting, at least for me, you trust this person not to do this. Even with Skype, when I was in France last summer, the girl that I was dating, we definitely had some Skype sex. There's that element to it. It's just as emotionally intimate as other sex is. I can't see myself doing that with any random girl. It's more like I am afraid that she might mention to someone else or something like that.

SEXUAL AND ROMANTIC STATUS

When I asked about future romantic relationships, Chandler said they "probably" would be with a woman. Only recently has Chandler begun to consider his sexual interest and romantic crushes on guys. Has he ever had a crush on a guy?

> I mean I've always romantically, I can't think back in high school where I was romantically attracted. Right now, there's this guy who lives in my dorm, and he's really talented and really smart. And he's open. He's a proud gay. And I'm in the closet. And he was talking a lot about his sexual experiences and how he always ends up bringing guys out of the closet by hooking up with them or whatever. I was attracted to that. And also because he's hilarious and supremely talented. And he's very comfortable with himself, which is another really big thing . . . I know I am never going to act on it.

> R: Have you ever had genital contact with a guy?

Mainly because if I was kind of alone with this guy that I was attracted to and there was no possible way that the outside world could know about it, I probably would do it. But I feel like for me the biggest thing is I am definitely more attracted to girls than guys. But at the same time, I am willing to experiment, and if I do experiment with a guy and girls find out they will look at me differently. And I don't want that. Differently in a negative way.

R: What if it was risk free?

I would definitely do it because I definitely am attracted to male genitalia. It is very stimulating for me. I don't think that I could openly just be gay. I don't want people to think of me differently. When I look at gays, I obviously really admire them, but I also look at them differently as opposed to if they were straight. I don't want that.

R: In your sexual fantasies, are they of males and females?

For me, it used to be all females, and then I participated in this group sex sort of thing. I think after that I was really a lot more attracted to guys than I would have been.

R: Did guys touch you?

No . . . This wasn't in college. This was in high school.

R: You've thought about your sexuality, and you're comfortable with it.

Yeah. It's more of an acceptance.

R: Have you told anyone about the nature of your sexuality?

Honestly, not at all. I actually have just not spoken about this at all.

R: Have you had the experience of a guy coming on to you?

Maybe to an extent to this guy that I am referring to. Again, it's sort of tricky because I was in a relationship . . . So like right now

> I have been dissociating myself from this entire thing. For the time being, I am asexual. I don't want anything to do with anything. It is tough.

Chandler is attracted to petite women, and breast size doesn't matter. "It's mainly just the curves and the body." For guys, it's more a matter of personality, of their confidence. "I am attracted to gay guys more than straight guys. If you are kind of out and totally gay and cool with it." Sexually, Chandler prefers guys to be physically feminine, not masculine.

MUSINGS

I asked Chandler if he believed that mostly straight guys exist. "Yeah, I feel like I am definitely one of those." If so, how does he differ from a straight guy? He noted two ways. "When I watch porn, I feel like I would be a lot more stimulated with the male genitalia. I have never watched gay porn, but when I do watch straight porn I definitely pay a lot more attention to that. That's one way. I feel like another way is maybe if I was totally straight I wouldn't really care so much about my masculinity. I feel like a lot of the times I got out of the way because I am insecure."

There weren't any out gay youths in Chandler's middle school or high school until his junior year. His parents are progressive in their attitudes toward homosexuality, but as best as he can determine there are no gays in his extended family. If not for his self-imposed limitations on his sexuality, which might have their basis on his perception of family and cultural prohibitions, would Chandler be headed toward bisexuality? He has the sexual and romantic attractions for men and has a special place in his life for male genitalia and feminine, confident gay guys, and he admits he should come out of the closet—but what closet and how far? For the moment, Chandler identifies as mostly straight.

Of the mostly straight young men I interviewed, those who reported both explicit sexual *and* romantic same-sex inclinations most stretched the boundaries of the mostly straight. This included not just Chandler but certainly Mike and Ryan and, to a lesser extent, Ben and Joel. Whether they will migrate toward bisexuality over the next several years I can't answer. Though I'm not sure where the boundary is between mostly heterosexuality and bisexuality, these young men are stretching it. They're doing it with their increased level of self-awareness, their openness to new experiences, their blend of sexual and romantic attractions to guys, and their sexual and romantic fluidity.

do mostly straight youth exist?

I think that even if you are straight and married to a woman you can still find men attractive. Maybe this is just me, but I feel like all men have at least one male-to-male experience in their life, whatever that [experience] may be.

(JONATHAN, AGE 23, GAY)

WHEN I FIRST INTERVIEWED the 160 young men in the Friends and Lovers project, mostly straight as a culturally recognized sexual identity did not exist. Four years later when I interviewed the forty-six young men in the Personality and Sexuality project, mostly straightness was beginning to permeate into the larger culture and the scientific literature.

Do young millennial men believe mostly straight men exist? Had they heard or read about them? Were they personally acquainted with any mostly straight men? Although straight and gay men had doubts about the existence of mostly straights, young men who are not exclusively attached to one sex or the other firmly believed that mostly straight youths were out there. Several knew a mostly straight man personally.

STRAIGHT VIEWS

Straight young men were largely unfamiliar with the term *mostly straight* and rarely knew anyone who so identified. Not unexpectedly, they largely doubted such guys exist. Perhaps, they questioned, such guys were, in reality, closeted bisexuals or gays?

- "I would think they were bisexual but a little bit afraid to admit it or to seek out that path because it's a little more embarrassing."
- "To me, it sounds like a guy that is just made uncomfortable by gay sex. That's what it sounds like to me at least."
- "The closest thing is that my friend thought he was bi when he was in middle school but he since changed to being heterosexual. But it wouldn't be too far from being bisexual."
- "I personally have never really thought about that. I don't really know what would drive someone to be that. I've never met anyone who claimed to be that."
- "I don't really understand how that would work. I don't know if it's a thing. I guess it suits being bisexual, but not to the same degree."

Some believed it was an "interesting idea," but it didn't apply to their life. Or did it? Several straight youths struggled with its possible meaning—if a man admired other men's bodies did this make him mostly straight? "No," one man quickly interrupted himself. "I have no sexual interest in other males."

- "I don't know. That's tough. I have been in the shower with guys for the last six years through hockey, and I am not sexually attracted to them, but you can still look at their body and say they are a sexually attractive person. I don't know. It's a tough spectrum. It's so hard to draw those lines. If I can't classify it for myself, I don't know how I would classify it for other people."
- "I don't know if I would put it to myself. I see how a guy could be attractive, and I have no problem acknowledging that. I just have no interest in doing anything physically or sexually with a guy."

It is important to note that straight men confined mostly straightness to the sexual and not the romantic realm. My guess is that the romantic domain might be perceived as dangerous territory because many straight young men have or have had quite strong emotional attachments with other guys. That experience would be much easier to normalize between young men than it would be to have sex with another male, even if it were a best friend.

I was pleasantly surprised with the relatively low level of disgust or negativity expressed by straight men with mostly straightness. Perhaps they could personally identify with having a slight degree of sexual attraction to other guys, or it just didn't affect—or threaten—them. As one straight guy simply stated, with a classic libertarian attitude, "I would feel just the way I feel about anyone else. Just normal. That is their preference. As long as it's not affecting me adversely."

With education and exposure, my guess is that straight guys will reconsider and probably accept the existence of mostly straight guys. But will they read the life histories of the guys in this book and understand? I'm not so sure, especially if they have strong, singular sexual and romantic preferences for women. All I would ask them to do is to consider whether some aspects of the mostly straight life resonated with their own experiences.

PRIMARILY STRAIGHT VIEWS

Perhaps not surprisingly given their small degree of same-sex sexuality, primarily straight young men strongly attested to the mostly straight phenomenon. Demetri was clear about this. "I don't think they are closeted gay people. I think they are primarily straight." Ricky recalled a couple of guys he thought might be mostly straight.

> In the same [way] that I wouldn't see it as possible for me to love another man, there are other people who love other men. It's another viewpoint. Who am I to say that you can't love both men and women? I can't do it. But I don't know if I would doubt the fact that you could do that. I feel like the 10 percent [same-sex sexuality] wouldn't be there unless it was the truth. I would be more inclined to believe that rather than 50/50 bisexual.

One young man acknowledged that invisibility likely handicaps the willingness of other young men to identify as mostly straight. "I think a lot more people would identity as being somewhere on the spectrum as opposed to just being on the extremes. Like I think myself, I would probably be towards the 10 percent just because it might be just because of my age now or just that I am very sexually open. I don't know."

BISEXUAL VIEWS

Bisexual youth were fervent believers in the spectrum of sexuality and of sexual fluidity, and thus had little difficulty imagining degrees of other-sex and same-sex sexuality coexisting. According to one bisexual young man, "Definitely they exist." Another succinctly summarized his take: "I think there is everything out there. I think there are probably people who have every level of attraction." Indeed, he thought he might be mostly straight during his early college years until he started dating a guy. At that point he felt he should probably identify his sexual and romantic fluidity as bisexual. None of the mostly straight men I interviewed has thus far dated a guy, though several were willing to consider doing so.

Many of the bisexual men I interviewed didn't believe that the vast majority of men were either totally straight or totally gay.

- "Going back to Kinsey, very few people are exclusively one thing or the other. And I do believe that. I can't discount that it's a real thing."
- "I am a believer in the Kinsey scale and the fluidity and everything like that. I actually think that there are people like that who are just open."
- "Well, I don't really believe in exclusive sexuality at all. I think exclusive heterosexuality is a myth to begin with. But I would say if that category does exist, I think that most guys that consider themselves exclusively straight would actually be in that [mostly straight] category."
- "I am more inclined to believe they exist than guys who are straight and have no attraction to other men exist. I am of the opinion that it is rare to find someone who is actually a 0 or a 6 on the Kinsey scale."

- "I don't know if that's a real or natural personality for people to have. I don't know if they are only 5 percent to 10 percent because of societal upbringings or if they are just biologically 5 percent to 10 percent. But I think if you're asking if these people exist in the world, then definitely. I think it's a continuum."
- "It's always hard for me to imagine that someone can be purely one side or purely the other. All people have different degrees of attraction."

One bisexual young man thought he understood why there might be disbelief that mostly straight guys exist. "I think a lot of people parade around as mostly straight. It's the same thing as like a lot of people come out as bisexual and just end up being gay. That's where people start to believe they don't exist. I haven't come across one yet, but that doesn't mean they don't exist."

By contrast, several bisexual youths had personal, convincing interactions with a mostly straight young man.

> They're not closeted gay people. I don't think anyone has enough self-control to override their sexual attractions. There are actually two or three guys that I am friends with that identify as mostly straight and have girlfriends, but there have been times where they say, "If only I were gay I would definitely do things with you," or that kind of thing. One guy, when he was drunk actually, he didn't try to kiss me but he was very forward, more so than any other heterosexual guy. I think it's more of a thing they haven't experienced before, and they aren't necessarily feeling completely fulfilled emotionally or physically with whatever situation they have with women. This is just me speculating, but it might be an outlet for them to feel that part fulfilled.

One young man believes that he has proof that mostly straights exist because he was "hooking up with one right now. He is mostly attracted to females. He's always been with girls. I just happen to be that one that he really liked. I was his first, and we still hook up to this day because we get along."

Critical for one bisexual young man was contrasting the "fake mostly straights" from the true types. For the phonies, he gathered his evidence from Grindr and Craigslist postings. Some guys say they're totally masculine and totally straight and "who are creepy, who do their masculine thing and say, 'Hey bro,' and 'I like to mess around occasionally.' People I suspect who are very closeted and will at some time come to terms with being gay." He distinguished the shams from those who are "like, yeah, definitely, mostly straight." Unfortunately, many of the true types are unwilling to be "up front about it, and if I find them they will tell you [they're] 'straight.'" He hoped this too would pass.

MOSTLY GAY AND GAY VIEWS

The gay and mostly gay youth that I've interviewed—whose stories can be found in my book *Becoming Who I Am: Young Men on Being Gay*—have had mixed views regarding the existence of mostly straight men. Ironically, given their small degree of attraction to women, *mostly* gay youths seldom gave their comrades on the *mostly* straight end of the continuum the same freedom to have a slight attraction to their less preferred sex (guys). And, aligning themselves with straight men, many of these mostly gay and gay men expressed significant doubt as to the authenticity of mostly straightness.

The gay and mostly gay youths who were most likely to grant that mostly straights exist can be broken down to two groups. If they had friends who identified as mostly straight, then they were more likely to consider the possibility of mostly straightness. For example, Jake's best friend in middle school was mostly straight, "with some same-sex attractions that it was never something he would have acted on." And after Raj joined a fraternity he discovered many of his brothers were, as they termed it, *bicurious*. He was less certain that they were attracted to men in the same way that he is, but he believed his brothers were saying that they "can enjoy sexual experiences with men."

The second group consisted of gay youths who were firm believers in the continuous nature of sexuality. If they judged sexuality was not simply a matter of being either straight or gay, then mostly straights must exist. Asher subscribed to the Kinsey scale, and he had friends who identified as straight, but if "they're horny and there's a willing guy, then why not?" Nicholas took a similar view: "I mean, I guess I haven't viewed it as a dichotomy. It's more of like a spectrum. It's totally possible to me." He, too, has met "some people that are that way." Rather than being horny, he noted, they wanted to do things with men they can't do with women, such as being a bottom.

Tyler and Jonathan also assumed that "anyone can fall anywhere on the spectrum," but for different reasons. Tyler considered that "it's wise for everyone to be able to experiment." If a guy wants to make out with a guy, he's labeled gay, and that's it. "And I don't like that. If someone wants to experiment to try to figure out what they like or if somebody wants to be mostly straight, let them be mostly straight." For his part, Jonathan didn't believe anybody can be truly straight. "I think that even if you are straight and married to a woman you can still find men attractive. Maybe this is just me, but I feel like all men have at least one male-to-male experience in their life, whatever that [experience] may be."

Yet I found these ostensibly open-minded views troubling when they failed to recognize mostly heterosexuality as a legitimate sexual and romantic orientation. Some gay youths were more willing to acknowledge mostly straight behavior than grant that a young man who called himself mostly straight could be describing an essential truth about his identity. If a guy is horny, wants to switch gender roles during sex, or experiment, then he might be mostly straight. It was as though it was only what happened in those moments that made a person mostly straight. Perhaps, they theorized, the mostly straight guy is afraid to do more with men because of what that would make him—gay. And several took the view of gay wrestler Reuben, who said in his vlog, "If you're a straight guy, and you let a guy suck your wiener, you're freaking gay, man, because, like, because you're getting off to that" ("Bromance," https://www.youtube.com/watch?v=jSPLofCU-Ks).

Geoff also assumed a negative view, that mostly straightness is only a momentary state of being, which leads him to discount the existence of mostly straight men. Rather, it's about straight men who "just get horny and want what they can get whether it's a guy or girl. I don't think it's an attraction. They're just looking for an orgasm or sex."

Dion hesitated before concluding, "Mostly, no. Maybe they do. But I feel like most of the time that's not the case."

> R: If they say they're mostly straight, what do you think they're saying about themselves?

> I think it's usually a number of things. One, people are saying it because they think it and it's a turn on for other guys, so it's not truthful. Or I think it's just they're socialized to think that gay is a bad thing or that being gay means that you act or are a particular way that's unfavorable. So they are straight, but they like guys.

> R: They may be gay guys under cover?

> Yeah! I mean I guess I do know a couple guys that I guess are mostly straight but sometimes they may hook up with another guy, but it's usually like a spontaneous kind of thing or with their girlfriends. Like they've had same-sex encounters but that's not how they identify or what they normally have and what kind of sex they prefer. So I do believe it exists. But usually that's not the case.

Lenny's dismissal was based on his belief that a "bromance" would rarely evolve into "Hey, I want to have sex with you." David could not relate to it either: "This is one of those complexes where I always say, 'Everyone sees different colors but doesn't realize it.' My green could be your red." So, too, Anthony considered such men as either "wanting sex with anybody or wanting to experiment and be different."

Of the gay men I interviewed, Ted was the most conflicted and thoughtful. He had greater confidence in the existence of sexually oriented than romantically oriented mostly straight men.

> I don't want to necessarily say if they exist. Those probably aren't the words I would choose. I would say, "Yes, that is a tendency at a particular time in their life." That is totally cool. I think that's definitely true.

> R: Can mostly straight be a lifetime orientation?

> I personally don't know because I don't know enough of them. I know quite a few of them. I think that some of them, I know my sperm brother [a donor-sperm sibling from a different family] is

one of them and says, "Well, I am mostly straight!" or "Well, I go both ways," or "I am only gay on Tuesdays," or whatever he says. And to me, I think that tends to be a little bit more of a physical thing than an emotional thing. I think for me a big part of being gay is, it's not just because I like to have sex with men, that's not the only part. I am never going to be able to love a woman the way that I love a man. I am never going to be able to look at a woman and say, "I am in love with every piece of you, not just your body. The way you move, the way you talk, the way you act, the way you behave, your construction, your mannerisms, the whole thing." It's a construct of a person, and I think the idea that somebody could be mostly straight disregards some of that. But I do think that there should come along a guy who says, "I don't know, probably for me." There may be 1 in 1,000 women that for me, I can say, "I love you." And I found one of them, but I can't love her the way I love a man.

BELIEF AND DISBELIEF

No surprise, all mostly straight young men emphatically affirmed that mostly straights exist. They contrast with the young men, especially the straight men, on the extreme ends of the sexual/romantic spectrum who expressed considerable doubt about the existence of mostly straightness. Few were willing to totally dismiss the possibility, but they had misgivings. Perhaps, they argued, a mostly straight man is simply a horny straight man willing to experiment because of his sexual or political beliefs. Or, they conjectured, he is simply a closeted gay man (similar to the view of vlogger Reuben) who wants to have gay sex without engaging the stigma of being homosexual in America. Saying mostly straight would then be safer, an easier out that would allow him to do what he desires, whether to test or to express his true sexuality.

Straight guys could rarely imagine why a straight guy would want to do anything with a guy, unless the man in question was confused about his sexuality or was in a situation where a woman wasn't available. Straight men might not be aware of another point that is in between themselves and mostly straights—the primarily straight men who are less straight than exclusive straights but who attest to having a slight amount of same-sex sexuality, less than mostly straight guys.

For their part, gay teens frequently recalled their own "bisexual phase" during the coming-out process when they resisted being totally gay by holding out "hope." They just assumed that being mostly straight is similar, a safe stopping over point on the way toward total gayness. As we now know, few mostly straight youth go down that path. If he is going to switch, then he returns to straightness.

In contrast to straights and gays are the bisexuals, who exist along the spectrum of sexuality but at different locations—whether primarily straight, bisexual-leaning straight, bisexual, or bisexual-leaning gay. They appreciate living one's life being "in between," so it's easy for them to imagine the possibility of being both less bisexual and less straight than other men.

It is noteworthy that after many "dislikes" were registered on his video, Reuben modified his original perspective about straight guys who have gay sex to something more in line with the nonexclusive guys in this book: "If you're a straight guy and you do something more than hugging . . . if it's like making out, or it's like a nice smooch . . . or anything beyond that, I personally feel like they're bisexual, they're not straight, they're gay, they're curious—they're not straight" ("Bromance Part 2," https://www.youtube.com/watch?v=EjVOl1EJslM). In this, Reuben leaves room for mostly straight guys.

In my view, the best proof of the possibility of mostly straightness is the fact that many adolescents and young adult men vouch for mostly heterosexuality as a real sexuality that is relevant for their life. This should be sufficient reason to believe mostly straight guys exist.

dillon returns

He is like older, maybe 30. It was a hookup, not like sexually, but to hang out, drink, eat, and talk. We kissed on the lips when we said goodbye. That was it.
(DILLON, AGE 22)

Sexual was still there. Just feeling comfortable and knowing someone and having them understand that. The most I ever did was make out.
(DILLON, AGE 27)

AGE 22

Slightly more than a year after the initial interview with the Friends and Lovers project, I sent a follow-up survey to those who had given me permission to do so. Dillon immediately responded. However, unlike everyone else, he requested an in-person interview because "a big thing happened in my life I have to tell you about." One of Dillon's friends lived nearby, so we arranged to meet in person when he came to town to visit him. And, since he was on campus, Dillon volunteered for an ongoing lab study in which we measured an individual's pupil dilation while he watched various sex scenes. We paid twenty dollars to all participants.

Having graduated college, Dillon, now 22, was employed as a human relations specialist for an automobile company with considerable travel obligations across the Northeast. But his new job was not the big surprise he wanted to share with me. I entertained other far-fetched, improbable possibilities: Will he announce he now identifies as gay? Did he find a romantic partnership with a guy? Or would this be a tale of a mostly straight guy turning totally straight?

The big announcement was none of these and, indeed, surprised me. In the last semester of his senior year, Dillon found "the person who I truly love and am committed to fully. Love is the most amazing and powerful feeling in the world. It hits you when you least expect it." With this love came the "most amazing, incomparable sex I've ever had with a girl I love." Dillon has given up his "brief flings" because he has his true love (a woman), wants to marry (a woman), and is having as much sex (with a woman) as he could ever want. With this Dillon launched into a lengthy detailed and excited history of their relationship.

Here's the abbreviated version: Dillon noticed a cute girl in a lecture course during his senior year, they locked eyes, she smiled, and Dillon listened for her name when exams were distributed. Facebook gave him more information about Maggie, and he arranged to surreptitiously bump into her at lunch ("I'm not like stalking her or anything. That's creepy."). Not wanting to immediately friend her, Dillon discovered on her Facebook page that she described herself as down-to-earth, level-headed, a wild child, and a field hockey player—an exact replica of what Dillon has been searching for!

As per his custom, Dillon invited several girls to a party hoping that at least one would show, and when multiples did, including Maggie, Dillon moaned, "I keep shooting myself in the foot!" Eventually, however, Maggie and Dillon became official after a special date in Central Park; they held hands, cuddled in a cab, marched for animal rights, and visited the Met to see an exhibit on Impressionism. One month later, they had sex, and now it meant something more than physical pleasure. "The word 'love' is on the tip of my tongue during sex, but I hold back because like I don't want to freak her out. A week later, we both say the L-word." What had formerly been his "most significant sex" now was usurped by Maggie. "I found the girl I want to be with for the rest of my life. Love came so naturally."

Dillon has an additional update: in his lifetime, "I've had eight intercourse partners, and I never came inside any until I did with Maggie. Not the first time but the second. It's never bothered me, and I've never had blue balls or anything." Dillon's priority has always been for the girl to get off. "I want her to shout, 'Dillon rocks my world, amazing sex, this guy did it!' With Maggie, it was the comfort level and our love that did it."

A third update, which now amazed me even more given what he just told me about Maggie, is that in the last year Dillon has gone out with a gay guy twice. These were not official dates but dinner outings. "He is like older, maybe 30. It was a hookup, not like sexually, but to hang out, drink, eat, and talk. We kissed on the lips when we said goodbye. That was it."

Clearly, Dillon was never your average straight hockey goalie. Yes, the beaming was still there, the softness, the eye contact, and the contradictory straight and gay dates. Dillon was having loads of sex with a woman he was considering marrying. Weighing everything, I expected Dillon to report on the questionnaire that he is now, irretrievably, totally straight.

After Dillon left, once again with multiple handshakes, I scanned the completed questionnaire he brought with him, and, consistent with previous reports, Dillon reported no sexual fantasies, sex, or romantic relationships with guys. However, despite his relationship and sex with Maggie, he maintained a slight degree of sexual attraction and romantic infatuation with guys. The sexual orientation label he selected was not "exclusively straight" but "mostly straight."

But what would the physiological pupil dilation data indicate? Dillon's eyes can't deceive, only reveal. Pupil dilation is an arousal measure below one's level of consciousness and thus cannot be manipulated or faked. True to his word, Dillon's pupil response to opposite-sex porn was consistent with straightness, even a little greater than the average straight guy. For same-sex porn, Dillon's eye dilation was in between straight and bisexual men—exactly where you would expect a mostly straight guy to score. On other measures, Dillon was slightly lower than straight men on adult masculinity, and higher on psychological well-being, extroversion, agreeableness, and conscientiousness. The last three indicate a pleasing personality—which I can attest to. On both self-report and physiological arousal measures, Dillon remains mostly straight.

AGE 23

Almost a year later, Dillon contacted me to say his work would be bringing him to the area and asked if I'd like to meet for Sunday brunch. Nicely dressed, looking the part of a junior executive with a corporate sweater with emblem, khakis, and moussed hair, Dillon had lost none of his magnetism or charm. He immediately apologized for not keeping in contact during the past year. We ate, he talked, and I took notes, with his permission.

Although Dillon and his girlfriend never got formally engaged, they were headed in that direction until jealousies surfaced when she went to graduate school on the East Coast and he was transferred to Chicago. They tried to stay together, but Dillon had difficulty trusting her, which he attributed to his father leaving the family. According to his side of the story, Dillon tried more than she did to make accommodations. Neither could relocate, and they separated several times, ultimately deciding it was not working. Dillon began having sex with waitresses and bar girls he met during his many travels.

Dillon's status was now 70 percent sexual attractions to women and 30 percent to guys. During his travels, he meets many gay men, and if they become friends they'll go to gay bars together, which doesn't bother Dillon. Indeed, Dillon admitted that he rather likes becoming a center of attention and pursued by gay men. He and his friends have talked on several occasions and rather openly about his sexuality. If ever he ever comes out, well, they would like to know. They're joking, but Dillon isn't. If he were to come out—but as what? Maybe he's bisexual, yet he doesn't feel the urge or motivation, despite the many opportunities to date and have sex with great guys. Although he wouldn't mind doing both, he'd rather go to a straight bar and pick up a woman for the night—which he does on many occasions.

Dillon's sexual fantasies are heavily populated with women. Although an occasional man appears, it's not frequent, intense, or central. I asked about his romantic attraction to his male buddies on one side and being "in love" with a guy on the other. Dillon says he's right down the middle. Consistent with his identification over the last three to four years, Dillon is more romantically mostly straight than sexually mostly straight, yet he is willing to try both. When I asked what kind of a guy he's attracted to Dillon named celebrities Patrick Wilson and Brad Pitt. The guy should be his height with blue eyes, blond, not too butch ("I'm not into bears") and not too femme, and should have an outgoing personality. In my notes, I wrote, "He just described himself."

AGE 27

Last summer, nearly five years after our last contact, Dillon, now 27 years old, texted me to arrange a time to catch up. Besides, he wanted to visit his old haunts on campus. We met in the same interview room as his first interview, and he gave me permission to record our conversation. "Sure, of course!"

Arriving 15 minutes late, for which he apologized twice with a huge smile, Dillon was clearly looking forward to this interview, which lasted nearly 90 minutes. He was no longer dressed as a junior executive; he wore blue jeans, a long-sleeve T-shirt advertising a craft beer, brown loafers without socks, a recent haircut (by his gay hairdresser), and a trimmed, short beard. Although he had gained a "little weight," he continued to work out (with recreational hockey). Dillon crossed his legs ankle to knee, had a firm handshake, talked with his hands, made great eye contact, and apologized several times for giving too many details or straying from the topic.

He and his almost fiancée have definitely, with acrimony, broken up, and they talk only on birthdays. She has a new boyfriend, and Dillon has a new girlfriend. Occasionally he longs to get back with his ex, but he has moved on. During the last five years, Dillon quit his human resources job, received a public policy master's degree on the West Coast, debated between several excellent job offers, and ultimately decided to enroll in business school, which he begins this autumn.

Although he and his current long-distance girlfriend have been together for over three years, Dillon does not see her as necessarily the "final one," though they've said the "love" word. The primary problem is one of location (she wants to be near her family), and in this they differ about where to live and work.

Although casual sex with women is once again less important to Dillon, he's uncertain that he's ready to give it up entirely. He's knows that his three-year girlfriend is "more serious than I am [he reviews her characteristics that irritate him]. She's been nice and loving, but I'm falling out of love, less attached." Plus, Dillon recently hooked up with a waitress/artist, and the relationship became intense:

> It just happened. Has ended but still there. Ended a week ago. Like two different lives, hard to describe . . . Glad I had this experience. She was 30 and very cool. She's from a different culture, more creative, big picture, visionary while I'm pragmatic. [I] loved it, this attraction, very strange. I knew [it] would be [a] transition period because of job and business school possibilities.

R: What is the understanding between you and your girlfriend in terms of sex?

> In terms of [me being] mostly straight, she doesn't know . . . My [gay] haircutter and I are very close, and she'll nag at me and say, "How is your best friend?" Not changed, don't think she'll understand. Saw him today and I like the flirtiness, and I like that but she hasn't seen that. [It's] so hard to explain to people.
>
> She knows I slept with lots of people, but she doesn't want to know that . . . out of sight, out of mind . . . I know she slept with five or six people. I probably don't want to know then or now. I don't think she's seeing someone on the side, 98 percent sure.

R: Are you attracted to men?

> Especially when I was in my job, [there] definitely was still an infatuation with guys, even more so. I had friends who are gay, and very good friends, and go to gay clubs with them. One friend older [than me] and we got extremely close, and sometimes we'd go to his place, make dinner, and cuddle and make dinner. I still had this aspect.

R: What was these gay friends' understanding of you?

> Pretty much "when are you going to come out?" I tell friends this is who I am and think it was hard for them to grasp at first.

R: Did you feel that if you had been willing to have sex the gay friends would have?

You know, at that point, I, possibly [because] it was still there . . . If you had to compare the percentages regarding relationships I would have said 60/40 to women to guys. It was just finding that right one. I would say romantic rather than the sexual. Sexual was still there. Just feeling comfortable and knowing someone and having them understand that. The most I ever did was make out.

One time [at a gay club] . . . this younger guy came up and I kissed him. [My friends] saw us and said we ought to go out, and their recollection was we were making out. No, we had kissed or whatever and wanted us to get close, and we exchanged numbers. He texted me for brunch. I didn't feel comfortable doing that, and our expectations were completely different. It was nice to have that . . . [My friend said] "You're probably gay or bisexual," and I said, "No."

[It's] hard to explain that I'm mostly straight, but people don't understand, thinking everyone is gay, bi, or straight, no in between. But this is how I feel. I think he understood it and wasn't something I always harped on. I think it'd be so difficult to go out and find a guy who was on the same kind of wavelength.

R: When you kissed the younger guy can you recall how you felt?

Probably it was fun. I didn't feel nervous, fine, pressure because could feel eyes behind my back. "We know he's seeing a woman and sleeping around with girls." So I felt pressure. Attracted to him but not aroused. Thought about actual sexual contact and it might get to that point, but at that moment I wasn't aroused. Nice to have.

R: When you go out with straight male friends how is it different?

Not the sexual pressure . . . I [find myself] less willing to talk about this. If [I] go out to [a] bar and [there's a] girl and guy I'd go toward the girl . . . Still there, physical attraction to straight male friends. Absolutely.

R: How do you see your future, sexually and romantically?

Right now, not into bar girls . . . If no girlfriend or if [we] break up, then definitely see myself going back to casual sex. Not as much but still be there. Would be smarter and not take myself off-track because have to do business school. Still very sexual.

Dillon has never heard of Josh Hutcherson or other celebrities who have come out as mostly straight. I asked if there have been any changes in his sexuality since his junior year of college. "No, but I forgot to tell you something my last year in Chicago." He had gone to a bar (not gay) and met a guy; they played pool, and the guy invited him back to his place for more drinks. There was no mention of sex, but Dillon began to wonder once they were there. Not feeling comfortable, Dillon left when the guy took a phone call. "Said to myself, nice exchange and nice guy. Didn't see myself going there. Came up so quick. Whole strangeness about his place and strange artwork he made."

Because Dillon brought the subject up again, I asked, "Where do you see yourself with sexual contact?"

[One] core friend, we've joked [about a] 3-way with a girl. With him I would if single, and in crazy days see myself doing that. We'll see, a possibility. Would only do things with the girl and not with him.

In terms of sexual contact with someone who wasn't a close friend, I don't know, but it'd have to be someone who could understand and be on the same wavelength because people are still rigid with gay, bi, or straight, and it seems that women have slightly more leeway in something in between bi and straight. It'd just have to be someone I feel more comfortable with, like my [gay] hairdresser because he'd be more understanding if we went out, but he's got a boyfriend and everything like that. He'd be someone who understands who is more my age. He's like 28 or 29. [I'd] go out with him, just the comfort level. Strange to say but I'm not opposed to going out with a guy and having that date, but then he'd say, "Where do we go from here?" We'd be romantic first and then have that part.

R: What if you knew that it'd be a one-time thing and no one would ever know? Just to have the experience?

It's a possibility. I wouldn't rule it out like never, just not that appealing to me. I haven't written it off, but if just [a] one-time thing, I don't know. If it happened to be someone I felt comfortable with, but just having that one-time thing, well, something about having that comfort, that connection. More likely to be one of my friends rather than a stranger, having that relationship is more important to me than a stranger. If [it] was a stranger and felt like I knew him forever even though you just met him at a bar, but I value the relationship more in that aspect versus a random hookup. But I'm not opposed to a random hookup if there was sex if it was the right moment and place.

R: Tell me more about the importance of your core group from high school.

Never give them up. Desire or need for male-male bonding and always important for me. I like that and something about having that, the brotherhood, the bond, mutual aid, tightknit, brotherhood I like, and longing for a relationship with a guy, especially with this group of guys. Hard for us not to get together. Go out, have fun, drink, slept in same bed, cuddling. Nice to have this and go back and crash with them and go to work. Still an excitement. Can't replicate that feeling [of] having this group of friends. Very fortunate to have it . . . Always keep contact with them.

Dillon emphasized how important it is to keep the bonding contact with his hometown friends—getting together with them endures for him as the best of times.

We say our good-byes, and Dillon gives me his permanent email address and the phone number he will always keep. Dillon wants me to remember that any time he's in the area, "if you want to follow up that'd be great. If anything comes up, then we can Skype or let me know." Dillon initiated a hug, we hug, and he's gone.

As a summary, the below chart should help you keep track of Dillon's sexual and romantic history (see Table 1). Several points are worth emphasizing.

· Dillon is incredibly stable in his mostly straight identity from high school to today (about a decade) into his idealized future.

Table 1. Dillon's sexual and romantic development

	Child[a]	Middle school[a]	High school[a]	Age 20[a]	Ideal future[a]	Age 22[b]	Age 23[c]	Age 27[d]	Ideal future[d]
Sexual orientation	Straight	Straight	Mostly straight	Mostly straight	Mostly straight	Mostly straight	Mostly straight	Mostly straight	Mostly straight
Romantic orientation	—	—	—	Mostly straight	Mostly straight	Mostly straight	Mostly straight	Mostly straight	Mostly straight
Sexual attraction to males	0%	0%	0%	20%	15%	5%	30%	15%	20%
Fantasy about males	0%	0%	0%	10%	0%	0%	5%	3%	5%
Genital contact with males	0%	0%	0%	0%	0%	0%	0%	0%	5%
Infatuation with males	15%	10%	10%	25%	20%	10%	20%	20%	20%
Romantic relationship with males	0%	0%	0%	0%	15%	5%	0%	0%	20%

a. Assessed at first interview for the Friends and Lovers project when he reported past and future.

b. Assessed at follow-up with interview and lab study.

c. Assessed informally at café discussion.

d. Assessed at 2016 interview.

- His same-sex infatuations have been present from elementary school, and they have consistently been the one domain that has nearly always been the highest in terms of the percentage directed to males. Guy infatuations, initially at 25 percent, decreased to 10 percent, and are now back up to 20 percent. Dillon has never been in a romantic relationship with a guy—though multiple candidates have appeared. In an ideal future, Dillon would like to date a guy.
- The most sexually erotic domains (fantasy, genital contact) have been nearly always been directed at females. For example, same-sex erotic fantasy, which was never high, he now describes as compromising 3 percent of his total fantasies.
- Dillon has never had sex with a man, only with women. He's had many opportunities for sex with gay friends and strangers, but he likes them not because they offer sex but because they provide romantic connections. However, in an ideal future, Dillon says he wants to have a same-sex experience.
- Sexual attraction has fluctuated the most, with the percentage devoted to guys wavering from 5 percent to 20 percent (now 15 percent). This inconsistency likely reflects the multiple ways in which Dillon uses this term, to reflect either sexual or romantic attraction, or both, and whether he is with a woman. Sexual attraction was low at age 22 because he had fallen madly in love with a woman and high at age 23 because they had broken up and Dillon was free to pursue casual sex.

developmental trajectories

Maybe I could say right now I'm 100 percent straight. But who knows?
In a fucking year, I could meet a guy and be like, "Whoa, I'm attracted
to this person." (JOSH HUTCHERSON, AGE 24)

WHAT MOST INTRIGUED ME during my interviews with the
mostly straight young men was their slight degree of same-sex
sexuality, which remained present without sacrificing their arousal
and desires for women. In this they differed from straight young
men. How can this be? Is it real?

Perhaps mostly straight men are simply more willing to acknowledge what some straight guys have but refuse to report—a
slight level of homoeroticism. Research has revealed millions of
straight guys engage in same-sex behavior and display romantic
attachment to other males. However, compared with straight
youths, mostly straight youths are more aware of their same-sex
sexuality, are less homophobic in their attitudes and values, and
are more progressive and hence immune to the social stigma sur-
rounding any recognition or expression of same-sex sexuality.
Hence, mostly straight youths are more likely than straight-
identified youths to *claim* their same-sex sexuality.

A second possibility is that mostly straight men differ from straight men not in their attraction to women or men but in aspects of their personalities. Perhaps what drives mostly straight guys to acknowledge their homoeroticism is their greater desire to experience new sexual situations, their greater curiosity about sexual matters, and their greater propensity for sensation seeking in all its forms. Hence, mostly straight youths are more likely than straight-identified youths to *pursue* their same-sex sexuality.

A third possibility is that the difference between mostly and exclusively straight young men is indeed hardwired—more a matter of nature than nurture. From this perspective, these are two different sexualities. Research shows that, like straight guys, mostly straight young men's genitals are aroused and pupils are dilated for naked female images. However, unlike straight guys, mostly straight young men have nontrivial increases in arousal responses to naked male images. They are, to use conventional terms, both heterosexual *and* slightly homosexual. They are not totally straight or gay, but rather are in between; to varying degrees they are considerably closer to heterosexuality than to homosexuality. Hence, mostly straight youths are more likely than straight-identified youths to *have* same-sex sexuality.

Another dilemma the life histories in this book raise is how mostly straight men differ from primarily straight men. We know the two share a similar sexual orientation—their pupil dilation to female and male images was nearly identical—and they have the same progressive social beliefs and levels of personal self-awareness. Yet mostly straight youths were at least five times more likely to report sexual attraction, sexual fantasies, sexual contacts, infatuations, and romantic relationships directed to other boys and men compared with the primarily straight youths. The largest and, perhaps, most critical difference between mostly straight and primarily straight youths was the willingness of mostly straights to engage in sexual contact with males—nearly 10 times greater, in fact. If these differences are not rooted in the biology of sexual orientation or progressive attitudes, perhaps they are based on personality differences. As I noted previously, mostly straight youths tend to be risk-takers, curious, and open to new experiences—such as sexual contact with males. They perceived, appreciated, reacted to, and pursued sexual and romantic opportunities more frequency than the primarily straight youths who, if they felt these emotions, pocketed them.

ARE THEY STRAIGHT?

The question before us is how best to make sense of the sexual and romantic lives of mostly straight, sexually fluid young men. Are they more similar than different from their straight brothers in their developmental milestones, from first sexual memories to how they envision their sexual and romantic future? A related question is do mostly straight youths follow a similar, singular developmental trajectory that diverges from that of straight young men? Or do mostly straight youths take multiple patterns, some of which are shared with straight youths?

These are tough questions to answer because we fail to grasp the developmental milestones of straight youths. It should be alarming—and embarrassing—that we as scientists understand so little about basic male sexuality and romance.

When it comes to straight male youths, in general we know the age of their first sexual experience, which is usually defined as vaginal/penile intercourse, a little about how well that experience goes, and perhaps a little about when they begin dating. We have adequate data on their age of pubertal onset, but we know little about the age of their first wet dream and their first masturbation. And we know next to nothing about their ages of first sexual memories, first crush, first experiences watching pornography, sex talks with parents, and first experiences with genital contact. For all of the above, with the possible exception of puberty, we know next to nothing about the straight guy's actual experience of these events: how he negotiates them, what he feels about them, and how they will impact his future sexual and romantic development.

I won't even attempt to fully explain why we know so little about these basic developmental milestones for the vast majority of straight-identified male youths. I will note, however, that being a straight male is seen as the default position, assumed unless proven otherwise. So scientists have often proceeded—falsely—as though straight men's lives do not need to be explained. By contrast, if a man constitutes "the other," then he's gay, and we do know a considerable amount about his developmental milestones— supposedly in contrast to being straight. As a result, I have a sense of how mostly straight youths differ from gay youths on some of these issues but not how they differ from their closer neighbors on sexual and romantic continuums, the straight youths.

Below I summarize the basic developmental patterns I saw across mostly straight young men, and when possible I compare these with those of their straight and gay brothers. Due to the incompleteness of our information, particularly about straight boys and men, at times I'll need to speculate or rely on some assumptions. If I could be allowed one request of my fellow scientists, it would be that we should ask straight male youths about their experience of sexuality and romance—not just about the age at which each milestone was reached but about the meaning and impact of each milestone on their life histories.

WHO ARE THEY?

The mostly straight, sexually fluid young men I interviewed hailed from diverse geographic regions of the United States, from many racial, ethnic, and religious groups and social classes. Nothing in this description is unique to them. They look a lot like the rest of America's teens and young men, including their straight and sexual-minority brothers. If you were to see a mostly straight or sexually fluid young man on campus, you wouldn't recognize him. On his person, there would be no "mostly straight" or "I'm fluid" symbols, no special clothing, rainbow colors, or stickers. On campus, there would be no mostly straight pride marches, mostly straight film festivals, kiss-ins among mostly straights, organizations fighting for mostly straight rights, resource centers welcoming mostly straights, peer empathy call-in centers for closeted mostly straights, or support groups to help mostly straights cope with microaggressions, fit in, or come out. Hell, he might not even recognize himself or others like him in classes, at work, on his team, in his fraternity, or at parties. There's no mostly straight community but also little profound discrimination against or rejection of mostly straights.

None of the young men have come out to their parents about their mostly straightness, and most remain closeted even to their best friends. Although most are living secret lives with a unique history and an uncertain future about how their mostly straightness will play itself out during their lifetimes, I join them in remaining uncertain about how their sexual and romantic status will influence their lives. At this point I see no evidence that the typical mostly straight male youth frets about his identity or is anxious, depressed, or consumed by his place on the sexual or romantic continuum. Whether he and other sexual-minority youths can learn from each other's experiences waits further evidence.

As this book is intended to present the mostly straight case, I will discuss what we know about the sexual and romantic development of the average mostly straight young man. I begin with his childhood and progress through the developmental milestones that likely occur during adolescence and young adulthood.

CHILDHOOD

As boys, nearly all mostly straight young men engaged in typical boyhood games and activities, usually with a small group of boys and one or two best friends, who were also boys. They played team and individual sports, especially soccer and cross-country, but also basketball, hockey, tennis, wrestling, and street games. Forts, swords, *The Three Musketeers, Star Trek, Star Wars,* and plotting against evil (including sisters) also occupied their time.

Some were leaders of their small group of friends, who were centrally located in their social group and quite popular. Others were loners, awkward, uncool, and invisible. Most fell somewhere in between for spending time with friends, some of whom remain best friends today.

They described themselves as masculine boys, though they differed in how they defined this concept and the degree to which they saw themselves as "man-wired." They could be competitive, masculine dudes, handy with tools, level-headed, calm, dirty, opinionated, tech oriented, and more rational than emotional. They also found ways in which they were feminine boys: a good listener, a talker, in touch with their feelings, artistic, and academically oriented. Several noted a higher degree of femininity during their childhood, such as having a preponderance of female friends, caring about their appearance, wearing strange clothing, and being called out as gay or weird. Several of the mostly straight young men stressed that their childhoods and adolescences were not "super macho." This descriptor was nearly always an anathema to them, reserved for their straight peers.

Both plentiful and persistent, girl crushes were recalled from an early age (preschool) through puberty, though what attracted them to a particular girl varied. Being pretty and athletic were bonuses, as were early signs of physical development such as "prominent boobs." Few told the object of their infatuation— or, for that matter, anyone else—with an occasional parent or friend exception. These crushes seldom evolved to sexual encounters, dating, or romantic relationships, though some remain friends today. If there were boy crushes, they were not recognized as such. Rather, they were best friends, buddies, or comrades. Only in retrospect and with little regret did mostly straight youths reinterpret what might have been going on as a boy crush.

Their first sexual memories were usually based on attractions to girls (female nudity, lady on a rug, *Playboy*) or sexual/erotic activities, whether sliding down a pole, French kissing a girl, or humping a blanket. In several situations, a first memory involved sex play with a boy, showing and touching genitals, or a pleasurable experience they understood as "wrong" but enjoyed nevertheless. Nearly all sexual memories were kept secretive until a much later age, including our interview. They would have been extremely embarrassed if anyone knew; indeed, reciting these memories today was not always easy and elicited blushes, laughter, faraway looks, apologies, and stutters.

I doubt if any of the above childhood descriptions would radically differ from what I would have heard from straight male youths. I suspect that straight boys' lives are also diverse, and I suspect that a small amount of femininity, friendships with girls, and sex play with other boys would not seem out of place among straight youths. However, on average, mostly straight youths were slightly less masculine than the average straight youth and quite likely slightly more feminine—that is, they had attributes and behaviors more typical of girls than boys. I'm only guessing on these assessments.

With confidence, I conclude without supportive data that the mostly straight boys were far more similar to straight than gay boys in these characteristics.

PUBERTY

The age range of pubertal onset was, as one might expect, broad, from 11 to 15 years, which is typical of most boys regardless of sexual orientation. The young men were frequently vague about recalling not only the exact age but also the event that clued them in that they were beginning puberty. The early markers were consistent with what we know occur early, such as pubic hair and peach fuzz. Several youths noted events that occur later in the process, such as deepening of the voice, chest hair, and muscularity, and events that are unrelated to timing such as erections and sexual attractions. Most early markers such as growth of the penis and testicles went unmentioned, except for one youth recalling his "balls dropping." Though these are true indicators of pubertal onset, they are frequently too gradual to be noticed.

In general, puberty was an elusive memory, and few recalled explicit thoughts, feelings, or evaluations about what was occurring. It was almost as if puberty commenced outside of a mostly straight boy's awareness. A few were disappointed with the results of the changes, but others were thrilled to "be a man." Regardless of when or what was developing and how each felt about it, one near universal experience was the silence of friends and family about what was happening to their friend, son, brother, nephew, cousin, or grandson. Perhaps they noticed his physical and sexual changes but didn't speak about them, give advice about them, question them, or celebrate them. In turn, a mostly straight boy seldom volunteered information or feelings regarding what he was experiencing. It was as if he had become a man, but in a hush.

These experiences were in direct contrast to the memories of many gay youths I interviewed who were keenly aware of their developing bodies and were either disgusted with what was happening or overjoyed with the aftermath. Many felt they were receiving what they were most erotically attracted to or wanted other boys to be attracted to. It also clearly demarcated their erotic fascination with other boys, which could be a good or bad thing for them depending on where they were in the coming-out-to-self process—certainly it was consequential.

One common experience of pubertal onset is wet dreams, recalled by about half of the mostly straight youths. This is similar to what we know about straight and sexual-minority youths. When wet dreams were absent, usually it was because the boys had begun masturbating at an early age. The few who recalled the seminal emission imagery linked it with their current sexuality. Though they might have been confused or felt they had peed in bed, few boys of any sexuality said that they were prepared for their first wet dream or described it as a memorable event. The exception was some gay youths who recalled their dream's male imagery and were thus alarmed about what it might mean for their future self.

Far more important to the mostly straight boy was discovering masturbation. Now he was in control of his orgasms and could repeat them on demand. How to do it was learned by accident (rubbing an erection, climbing a pole, sitting in a Jacuzzi), or after hearing his friends or brother joke about it, or by discovering instructions on the Internet—by which he meant porn. Regardless, a mostly straight young man as a boy, like his straight friends, quickly learned the value of porn to enhance the motivation to masturbate and to increase its intensity. He also promptly learned to erase his computer history. Masturbations were generally frequent, perhaps once or more daily, and were positive experiences hidden from parents and seldom discussed with peers.

Porn watching, which many adults assume is fraught with overwhelming negatives, was frequently perceived as irresistibly positive by these young men. For example, porn was the major sex educator for boys, regardless of sexual orientation. Most began early, usually as puberty was commencing, and online porn became a frequent source of entertainment and inspiration. Porn was fun and energizing, though several of the young men noted it enhanced their misconceptions about sex and became a source of preoccupation and, occasionally, guilt.

Porn also served as a critical barometer of same-sex sexuality for mostly straight young men. Perhaps they noted the penis or the muscular enhancement of male actors, comparing them with their own. Whether they did this more frequently than straight boys, I don't know, but undoubtedly they were less erotically enchanted or obsessed with the male physique than were gay teens.

Likely consistent across youths of all sexual and romantic orientations, school-based sex education classes were usually only helpful in teaching a boy about the biology of pubertal changes and how to practice safe sex—that is, to abstain from sex. No one reported receiving instructions in class about how to masturbate, what are pornography's benefits, how to talk to girls about sex, what to do and expect when having sex, how to decide whether to have sex, how and when to ask for sexual consent, or what is the meaning of sex. Information about these concerns resided, whether rightly or wrongly, either on the Internet or in conversations with friends and occasionally brothers.

For sex and romantic information, almost none turned to parents. Only a few received—or wanted—helpful material or advice from parents. If parents tried to have a sex talk (and few parents initiated such conversations), it was too little, too late, and too wrong. How late was it? For several it was just before going away to college. What was the message delivered? Regardless of what the youth had done, was currently doing, or planned on doing, the counsel was something akin to "don't do anything stupid," "don't sleep with dirty girls," and "use condoms."

PUBERTY IN PERSPECTIVE

Are mostly straight youths typical in these pubertal matters? Yes, they were nearly identical with the national norms for age when reaching biologically based events and the percentage who had a wet dream (about half) and masturbated (all). So, too, they seldom received adequate information from school-based sex education programs and had to rely on the Internet for sex knowledge, especially porn, during their developing years.

We know that parents can make significant contributions to an adolescent son's positive sexual experiences by enhancing his self-esteem, which is a critical factor for how adolescent sexuality is played out. How can they do this? Primarily by fostering an ongoing, high-quality relationship with him. That is, parents are important, yet too many evade their parental responsibilities by ignoring their son's physical and sexual development. This appears to characterize most parents regardless of their son's sexuality. Most parents are silent, tardy, or ineffective (not always, but frequently) in talking about what will happen during puberty and the mechanics and joy of sex.

Several differences separated the mostly straight young men from the gay youths I interviewed. Gay youths recalled, often with detailed, emotionally evaluative observations and judgments, their pubertal development—largely because these changes were linked with what puberty sensationalized for them. Puberty eroticized and gave new meaning to their same-sex sexuality, which heightened their awareness that they were at odds with their peers and perhaps with what they wanted at the time for themselves. As a result, the typical gay youth was quite attentive to his biological changes in terms of when the transformations began. He had explicit memories of genitalia growth and development, the effect they had on his body and sexual feelings, the imagery of his wet dreams and masturbations, the value of porn in helping him to define his sexuality, and how he felt about what was happening to him.

I saw little evidence that mostly straight youths mimicked gay youths in these matters, even those who had a significant degree of same-sex sexuality. Perhaps their overwhelming heterosexuality helped them feel typical among straight boys in general and kept them from feeling threatened by their slight homoeroticism. Consequently, they were not so keenly aware of puberty and its impact on their life.

Regardless of their sexual or romantic orientation, young men in our society live in silence during these years because they do not and cannot share what could be a rewarding, magical process. We can do better.

DATING AND SEX

Several mostly straight young men began serious dating in middle school—eighth grade was popular. Others never dated in high school but instead waited until the first year or two of college. The clear majority, however, began in high school, like their straight peers. Those who started early gained social prestige, but the relationships themselves could be unpleasant. Those who started late admitted to being somewhat socially awkward, shy, or introverted. The first dating relationship usually lasted several months, some even for years—two dating couples maintained their relationships for nearly five years. Long-term relationships usually ended once the two partners went to separate colleges or work locations. The practical limitations of maintaining a long-distance relationship were too tricky or challenging, or one or both simply wanted to try something different.

Sex among early dating couples often progressed no further than kissing and making out, though those that endured long enough to eventually include some level of genital contact, usually a hand down the pants, genital rubbing, or fingering. Oral sex was common for the couples who lasted multiple months. It was relatively rare for these initial dating relationships to advance to intercourse, although one young couple had intercourse on their second date.

Other than early child sex play among boys or occasionally with a girl, the first genital contact could be as young as 12 or 13 or as old as the early twenties. The most common ages were 15 to 17, with first intercourse around 17, though several of the young men entered college as virgins (no penile/vaginal intercourse). This status usually didn't last long, as the right woman or the right opportunity materialized rather quickly. Two young men preserved their virginity—one for religious reasons—at the time of the interview.

The first sexual partner often was a friend, who might later become a dating partner or a current girlfriend. Seldom was it a stranger. Having heterosexual sex was usually a multiple-time event, continuing within the context of what friends did together or what they believed was supposed to occur within a dating relationship. The first experience with intercourse was frequently problematic; seldom was it a great physical or psychological experience. It was an awkward moment for the mostly straight youth because of his inexperience or self-doubt or because of adverse circumstances: a condom leaked or didn't fit, a penis seemed too small or too big, erections were lost, or foreskins failed to retract. He eventually had an orgasm, but whether she did was usually unknown (but he suspects not). My best guess is that these experiences happen to straight youths at about the same level of frequency and frustration.

Many of the mostly straight young men have had a serious romantic relationship, and several reported experiencing true love with a girl or woman. In several situations, the couple contemplated marriage. Breaking up was nearly always difficult, and the reasons to do so were many (inadequate sex, personality conflicts, moving) and psychologically painful.

The young men provided little evidence that their parents knew, or wanted to know, about the extent of the sex they were having, especially if they were young or if premarital sex violated family values. Their friends might have known about the relationship, but in general there was little sense that either parents or friends were particularly helpful to mostly straight youths in navigating these relationships. Sons almost never went to parents for advice, and parents almost never offered to help their son, thus delivering the message "We don't want to know."

In terms of their future, nearly all mostly straight young men foresaw a long-term, monogamous relationship or marriage, usually by their early thirties. Their twenties was the best time to experiment with casual sex, both for pure pleasure and finding ("test-driving") the right woman. Comparable to gay youths, mostly straight young men were often more invested in finding their soul mate than in chalking up the numbers. Monogamy rather than an open relationship was the future desire for most, but not all, young men. Later, they might change their mind, but they weren't anticipating that they would.

Whether these patterns of dating and having sex are common among straight youths is unknown. Their age of first sex appears normative, as does the identity of the first sex partner: a girl they know because they're friends or dating. Although I do not know how long first relationships typically last for straight or mostly straight youths, the variety among the latter was impressive and likely normative.

SEXUAL AND ROMANTIC STATUS

None of the mostly straight youths I spoke with had yet had "real sex" (anal intercourse) or formed a romantic relationship with a guy. Several were willing to exchange blow jobs, but as best as I could tell only one mostly straight youth had yet given or received a blow job from another guy. Two had pre-pubertal sex play with another boy (and seemingly enjoyed it), two had genital rubbing and mutual masturbation sessions (also pleasurable and understood as "normal" boy things to do), two had another male touch his penis (without orgasm), and four made out with a guy (with or without alcohol). None classified a relationship he had with another guy as a dating situation, although many of these relationships had the characteristics of two people who are dating or in love (time spent together, emotional involvement, sharing lives, cuddling).

Nearly half have had or currently have gay guys hitting on them, which they tend to interpret as flattering rather than obnoxious. Regardless, the vibe given off by mostly straight men occasionally led others to suspect they might be gay, and not always only by gay youths. One girlfriend suggested a threesome with another male, one young man has been present for group sex with multiple guys present, and a girlfriend and parent said it was okay for the mostly straight youth to explore his gay side. Several mostly straight youths were enamored with the penises of porn stars or wished they were as jacked as the men they were watching. Others were attracted to "pretty" or feminine men, not to masculinity. These occurrences were likely, for the most part, to be more prevalent among mostly straight than straight youths.

Many mostly straight young men found men attractive (even "hot"), admitted to having bromances from an early age, and now understood some child and adolescent friendships as having been infatuations. One said he and his best friend "emotionally kissed." These romantic attractions and situations were more difficult than sexual encounters to label as "gay-like" because they appeared to the young men to be normative among buds. That is, it was more standard and customary to love your best buddy than to have sex with him.

Many of the young men reported they are now or have been "bicurious," "sexually fluid," or on the "bisexual spectrum." Several wondered if they might be bisexual or moving in that direction. Most would not be horribly averse to "trying out" sex with a guy, though few believed they would conduct an experiment with it now or in the near future. Their focus was primarily on women—as in, why take the lesser when you can get the real thing?

I can't predict the direction these young men will take once they reach full adulthood. Will heterosexual marriage, children, and a career take the oomph out of their same-sex curiosity? What exactly will happen to their small degree of same-sex sexuality? Will it fade into a distant memory or even oblivion? Will they have the occasional same-sex fling or develop intense friendships with other men? If Dillon is any indication, mostly straightness will not become obscure. He does not, however, yet provide guidance regarding how mostly straightness will eventually play itself out. I'll ask about this the next time Dillon checks in.

My best guess is that the mostly straight young man will continue to be an extremely progressive individual when it comes to sexual and romantic issues and that he and perhaps his wife or female partner will know about his sexuality and romantic nature. Perhaps it'll be their secret, or they'll share it with others.

if you believe you are mostly straight

[It's] hard to explain that I'm mostly straight, but people don't understand, thinking everyone is gay, bi, or straight, no in between. But this is how I feel. (DILLON, AGE 27)

IF I WERE TO MEET YOU, there wouldn't be any particular thing—not your body, not your look, not your personality—that would reveal to me your sexual or romantic orientation. At least when mostly straight young men walked into the interview room, I couldn't tell. Although they occasionally pinged a tiny bit of my gaydar, more often than not I was quite surprised when they announced, "I'm mostly straight." My guess is that you would be the same.

HOW CAN YOU TELL IF YOU'RE MOSTLY STRAIGHT?

Perhaps the easiest way to understand where you are along a sexual or romantic spectrum is to ask yourself about your attractions. What percentage is devoted to each sex? Has this changed over time or does it change depending on the situation? These percentages do not necessarily imply acting sexually or romantically on these attractions. You can be mostly straight and remain a virgin, without sex or love. Although engaging in sex and romance is a choice you make, your degree of erotic and romantic attraction to women and men is less under your control. As Dillon's life illustrates, these two may not always run in parallel, and this is certainly true for the clear majority of mostly straight men. Their lives lend support to a perspective that acknowledges—and embraces—sexual and romantic fluidity.

To be clear, Josh and Dillon can appreciate men sexually or romantically, but they value women even more and will likely have life trajectories that include marrying a woman and living a lifestyle that may be indistinguishable from a straight one. But what about you? Where do you fit on the spectrum?

As is apparent from the stories of mostly straight youth that you've just read, mostly straight men are diverse—physically, psychologically, and socially. Even in your sexual and romantic life you might not necessarily share the same degree of desire, arousal, sexual behavior, and public and private identity as another mostly straight youth. You should remember that just as there are tall people and short people with gradations in between, so, too, nuances exist along sexual and romantic continuums.

But if mostly straights are not of one kind, how can you figure out whether you're mostly straight? One strategy is to answer a set of questions. If you agree with one or more of the answers on the list below, you're a candidate for mostly straighthood.

1. What is your sexual identity? "I'm mostly straight."
2. Who are you sexually attracted to? "I'm almost always attracted to women, but on some occasions I'm slightly attracted to men."
3. In your erotic fantasies—say, during masturbation—what sex do you imagine? "Mostly women but sometimes a man enters the picture."
4. Who do you have sex with? "Almost always women, but I have or am willing to go some distance with particular men."
5. Who do you have crushes on? "Almost always women but sometimes men."
6. Who do you have romantic relationships with? "Almost always women, but I'm open if the right guy shows up."

But what does "slight" or the "right guy" mean? There's no consensus. Is it 1 percent, 5 percent, or 10 percent of your total? At what point is it so large (15 percent?) that it's more accurate to say you're along a bisexual spectrum? How many of the five dimensions (sexual attraction, sexual behavior, erotic fantasy, infatuation, and romantic relationship) must be covered, and is one more important than the others? Definitive answers are difficult to come by, but Dillon and the guys in this book should help you figure it out.

If you believe you might be or you're certain that you are mostly straight, both scientific research and the young men you've just met attest that *mostly straight* is a sincere and experienced sexual and romantic identity. Heterosexuality with minor same-sex sexuality has likely existed throughout history and across all cultures and before your own birth. It is who you have always been, even before you became aware of the meaning of your mixed sexual and romantic attractions. And there are millions like you, who share your sexuality. Now, at last, with the visibility of mostly straightness catching up with its reality, you can apply a name to your sexual identity.

IN WHAT WAY ARE YOU MOSTLY STRAIGHT?

Although I organized the book to reflect diversity among mostly straight adolescents and young men based on their sexual and romantic inclinations, this is not the only or necessarily the best way for you to understand your life.

First, our understanding of mostly straightness may change as scientists gather more information about the long-term trajectories of people's lives. Perhaps it is the *stability* or lack of stability of a mostly straight identity that is most critical for you. For example, you might be extremely stable in your identity, like Dillon who has identified as mostly straight for the past decade, or you may be more fluid, fluctuating among sexualities over time or circumstances.

Second, you might move between heterosexuality and bisexuality based on conditions or circumstances that we know little about. Is it meeting a guy who knocks you out with his personality, intellect, philosophy, or body? Is it a perspective, a book, a class, or an idea that creates a space for you to potentially love or to desire sexual union with a guy? If so, you might be willing to accept a new identity for yourself to better reflect the complexity of your sexual and romantic life.

A third possibility is to base distinctions among mostly straight young men on the *intensity* or the *frequency* of their same-sex attractions. Perhaps the most critical difference between you and a straight young man is not in the proportion of your total attractions, fantasies, and infatuations devoted to men versus to women but how often you have these various feelings and, once experienced, their intensity. Are they mild or severe, an occasional blip in your life or all-consuming, seldom or present during most of your waking moments? Are the feelings soft, worthy of a slight smile, or passionate, so thrilling that you have a difficult time distracting yourself? Are they merely an occasional bothersome moment or an unsettling theme of your everyday life?

A fourth critical decider might be *when* you experience your marginal same-sex sexuality. Is it only when you are drunk, high, or otherwise in an altered state of mind? Or is it simply as you go about your daily life, whether alone or with others? Does it take a significant visual, tactile, auditory, or aromatic stimulus to bring the attractions to conscious awareness?

A fifth possibility that would help you figure out what you are all about would be to distinguish whether you desire or are willing to act on your sexual and romantic attractions or whether you are content to merely have the sexual and romantic attractions and fantasies in the abstract. Is being sexual or romantic with another guy a passing thought, a hypothetical notion, or a fleeting think piece? Or do you actively and purposefully place yourself in situations to make it happen? If you want to make eye contact with a guy at a fraternity mixer, on the athletic field, a coffee shop, or a political club meeting, then the possibilities for enacting your same-sex sexuality and romance are greatly enhanced. Or you may be willing to satisfy your curiosity if the right guy comes along—if it feels safe and right for you, you'll go for it.

To expand on these distinctions, maybe it's falsely splitting hairs, but it feels important to consider separately those of you who engage in sexual or romantic behavior (genital contact, dating) from those of you who have erotic feelings and thoughts (fantasies, crushes) but no intent to express them behaviorally. Maybe this is what keeps you up at night or what inspires your sexual and romantic self. Certainly, what you do in terms of sex and dating is far more under your conscious control and is hugely susceptible to real—or what you perceive to be real—pressures to conform to socially desirable ways of being. This is especially pertinent during your teen years when you likely feel the heaviest burden to conform to the conventional wisdom of what it means to be either a straight or gay youth.

Of course, I'm not sure we should even care how you arrive at your decision because the critical piece is feeling authentic to your true self. If you have an unsettled identity that best fits where you are currently, why should anyone tell you or want you to be otherwise? Just listen to your heart. What is happening in your head need not ever be expressed by you or be known by others. It's your secret to keep if that's what you want, to judiciously reveal to a select few or to shout on Facebook. Whatever you choose, please be smart about it. Make sure that what you say and do fits with how you want your life to be.

In this regard, you are likely to be affected by nonsexual and nonromantic factors, such as lifestyles you might or might not want to follow, the attitudes and values of those you respect, and families and social networks you care about and must live with. Of course, others can't always believe who you are having sex with or dating adequately represents all of your reality. You can certainly date and have sex with the gender you are not erotically attracted to, and you can have a sexual identity that doesn't reflect the nature or the complexity of your sexual and romantic orientations. And these can change, which is the magic of sexual and romantic fluidity. It takes time and effort to sort through these things, which is fine. There is no rush. Used with good judgment, curiosity can be a blessing and add considerable excitement and clarity to your life. It's also true that patience and good judgment in these matters are always assets in making decisions. It's important not to feel locked in or feel that you must be consistent with previous conceptions of yourself.

ARE YOU ON A SPECTRUM?

As a mostly straight, sexually or romantically fluid youth, you have the option to either question or forego altogether the traditional three-category system—straight, bisexual, or gay. You can decide that you're "something else." Others, me included, may have no idea what you mean, at least until you talk about it—and that's okay. Although some straight and gay youth view you and your mostly straight brothers as horny or experimental straights or as closet cases destined for full gay membership, attitudes can change and are changing.

I hope you counter these simplistic notions of your straight and gay brothers with the perspective that sexual and romantic orientations are linked in a continuous manner with many points between the exclusive female/male attraction ends of the continuum. Sex and romance are a spectrum. If you believe this, then you're in sync with the young men I interviewed about the reality of their lives. They simply do not neatly fit in with our tidy, clearly marked sexual identity boxes.

If we acknowledge the reality of mostly straightness, this explodes the myth of sexual categories. It also implies that there are likely other identities along the continuum that we should learn about. To gay and straight people who still doubt this conclusion, I point to the scientific evidence (see Appendix B) that firmly establishes mostly heterosexuality in terms of physiological arousal, prevalence rates, reports of sexual and romantic indicators, and stability over time. Being mostly straight is a meaningful, bona fide self-description of an individual's sexual and romantic self—maybe your own or someone you love.

Male sexual fluidity is seldom on our radar screen, but it should be. It is not just women who are sexually and romantically fluid. Men, as you know, are as well. Perhaps your life reflects the basic evolutionary biology of our history that reinforces male-male bonding and slight but meaningful femininity in men. The ultimate message you as a mostly straight youth delivers is that to ignore the complexity of sexual and romantic desires denies us the ability to appreciate your life. To assume all straight men are equally, intensively, and frequently attracted to women shortchanges them and disregards the mosaic of their experience. We need not obscure your life by assuming you must occupy a singular category.

ARE YOU PRIMARILY OR MOSTLY STRAIGHT?

Given that primarily straight and mostly straight are sexual identifications and not necessarily based on the number or degree to which you endorse sexual and romantic indicators, it is noteworthy that primarily straight young men have reported a lower level of these markers compared with mostly straight youth. The primarily straight young men I interviewed averaged half the number of these sexual and romantic indicators compared with the mostly straight men, and as such their degree of same-sex sexuality is quite small, usually less than 3 percent of their total. Relatively few have ever engaged in sexual activities or had a romantic relationship with a man. It is, after all, easier to maintain an authentic membership in the straight world if your same-sex sexuality is felt through abstractions rather than behavior.

If you consider yourself to be primarily straight, you'll likely compare yourself to the straight and mostly straight points along a continuum. You could argue that you are simply more sexually and romantically fluid or inventive than your straight brothers. Because you tend to be ultra-progressive when it comes to sexual rights, this leaves you room to be flexible in your sexual and romantic life—even if you are just as straight as a straight guy. Saying you have a small degree of same-sex sexuality might place you exactly where you politically and socially want to be. In most respects, however, everything I've been saying to the mostly straight young man could also apply to you.

From another perspective, because you are fundamentally primarily straight this might well bolster your ability to see the world through a different lens, encouraging you to be more broadminded and accepting of those who are sexually and romantically different from you. And because you have this small degree of same-sex sexuality, you emit a vibe that gay guys, using their highly tuned gaydar, notice. Sensing you to be a super nice and attractive guy, they might be sufficiently delusional to hope they can pull you away from your heterosexuality. Receiving this undue interest from a gay youth, you'll likely refuse because that's not you, but you do it in an extremely supportive, nice manner: "Thanks, but no thanks. You're a very attractive dude, and if ever I hooked up with a guy, you'd be the one! You must work out a lot. What gym do you belong to?" I seriously doubt your straight friends give off this same aura, and if they were mistaken for gay, they might not be as nice as you would be in response to such overtures (though they should be).

Some young men in your generation might argue that if today you are primarily or mostly straight then tomorrow you'll shuffle along the spectrum toward bisexuality. If this were to happen, it would not be inconsistent with several of the primarily straight young men I interviewed who experienced your degree of fluidity as a weigh station before transitioning to a higher degree of same-sex sexuality. But is this shift temporary or permanent?

If it were truly your fluidity playing itself out, then these persistently recurring transitions would be expected and likely be momentary. If, however, these moves were to solidify, then they would reinforce your primarily heterosexual sexual orientation as a stable spectrum point in between exclusive and mostly heterosexuality. Some of the young men in this book gave up or minimized their small degree of same-sex sexuality and returned to a straight status; others enhanced their same-sex sexuality and moved toward mostly heterosexuality. You might do either, or it's also possible for you to stay put because it is where you should be. I can't predict which option will characterize your developmental trajectory.

Whether you move toward or away from exclusive heterosexuality might depend on the extent to which you are under the influence of *homohysteria,* which is apparent in some corners of our society—perhaps including your family, school, work, or community—and perhaps yourself. Although sexual prejudice is declining in your generation, it is not totally absent, especially in particular regions, classes, ethnicities, and political or religious groups. Lifting cultural restraints on acceptable forms of masculinity and sexuality would encourage not only your nonexclusive nature but also that of millions of other teens and young men who want to express their true nature as well so that they can better thrive in other areas of their life. Whether this trend will continue to inspire a growing number of straight youths to declare their small degree of same-sex sexuality as meaningful is an unknown. If this were to transpire, I believe we would discover that there are as many sexually and romantically fluid men as women. How large this number will prove to be is anyone's guess.

What we must do now is to listen to you and other young men like yourself. Are you a variation along a common theme or are you sufficiently distinct to consider you as an adjacent neighbor to straight or bisexual men on a sexual and romantic spectrum? Perhaps it doesn't matter because at this point both could be true.

ARE SEX AND ROMANCE THE SAME THING?

The life narratives of primarily and mostly straight young men provide one answer to the question of whether sexual and romantic orientations are the same thing. You can't assume they're identical. They're "kissing cousins"—related but different. Your sexual and romantic desires likely overlap such that the gender you prefer to have sex with is the gender you prefer to fall in love with. Or this might not be true for you. If you're mostly straight you might well be romantically and sexually attracted to women and men to varying degrees. Perhaps you only desire sex with women but occasionally find yourself falling in love with a guy, or you only fall in love with women and occasionally express your sexual feelings with men. Even your straight friends might enter the fray to confuse matters. One straight young man I interviewed answered my question as to whether he has experienced true love with "Yes, with my best friend, Sean."

If you give primacy to your sexual rather than your romantic attraction, would you miss what might be most interesting about yourself? If you were to do this, is there the possibility that you would not know the nature of your sexual and romantic worlds? I certainly would not have understood Dillon's life, which teaches us the value of giving priority to the full spectrum of sexual and romantic feelings, thoughts, and behaviors.

One straight young man told me during his interview that he *allows* himself to have sex with other men, but he dismissed it as a meaningful statement about his sexuality because it only occurs when he is under an altered state of consciousness (drunk or high). He identifies as straight because during orgasms he imagines women. Another straight young man argued that the significance of his same-sex experience depends on the type of sex he has—receiving oral sex has no impact on his sexuality, but receiving anal sex would.

Regardless, as should be obvious to you by now, there are no universal benchmarks in determining the relevant degrees of sexual and romantic indicators for your distinctive life narrative. The inevitable inconsistencies within heterosexuality might well confuse you, as it certainly does many of us. If you were subjected to physiological measures of pupil dilation, genital arousal, or brain imaging—which you would have little control over and couldn't manipulate to register what you want them to—perhaps a critical component of your sexuality and romantic inclinations would be clarified for you. Whether such information is consistent with your self-reports might depend on how aware you are of your sexual and romantic status or whether you have reason to deceive others or yourself. Clearly you can be exclusively heterosexual, primarily heterosexual, or mostly heterosexual based on your own idiosyncratic reasons.

SHOULD YOU COME OUT?

From my vantage point, few young men have come out as mostly straight—except in interviews and on anonymous surveys. Because the degree of same-sex attraction that you as a mostly straight youth feel is so slight, during adolescence you can ignore it or keep it a secret, likely without consequence psychologically or socially. You may have your excuses and rationales for its expression in your sexual behavior or its presence in your mind in the form of erotic or romantic fantasies. No one will likely ever know you're mostly straight unless you disclose this fact. You won't likely face social ostracism, biphobia, homophobia, or sexual prejudice of any sort. And if you should act on your fantasies sexually through an encounter with another guy or romantically by having a crush on him, both you and your partner might not share the same understanding of what just happened or how you feel about the intimacy.

If you do *not* come out as mostly straight, you should ask yourself whether you are running the risk of not being fully true to yourself. Should you be forthright about your same-sex desires? To pretend or to act against your nature likely costs you some degree of psychological well-being. You have the choice of whether to acknowledge your attractions and identify accordingly, as Josh and Dillon have. Josh is out to the world; Dillon is only out to some of his closest friends.

It'll take some explaining on your part, which can be quite awkward and perhaps consequential. Telling a male friend that you have a crush on him could threaten your friendship or mislead him into believing you are in the closet. You may lose him altogether if he is unable to accept your sexual and romantic reality. Of course, it's possible that your friend is also a sexual minority and is perfectly okay with what you tell him. Alternatively, if you are both unaware of mostly heterosexuality, the two of you may continue to understand your feelings for each other as normative of young men—without reference to sexual or romantic desires.

The question of why mostly straight youth don't declare their sexuality in this new world of sexual fluidity and acceptance is perhaps best answered with another question: What do you have to gain by coming out? Certainly, declaring any ounce of same-sex sexuality is risky. It is not universally seen as a positive—at least, not yet. So my answer to you has two parts:

1. Coming out as mostly straight likely contributes to your personal authenticity.
2. Coming out might well change the world—moving it closer to embracing same-sex sexuality in its many forms and degrees of expression.

QUESTIONS I CAN'T ANSWER FOR YOU

The young men I interviewed provoked additional dilemmas and questions I'm still not certain I can answer for you with much confidence:

- How much of a particular sexual or romantic indicator is necessary to tip the balance away from exclusively hetero-sexuality toward primarily or mostly heterosexuality?
- How frequent or how intense does your same-sex sexuality need to be for you to label yourself as not exclusively straight?
- Is any one indicator more telling of your primarily or mostly straight status than others?
- Sexual attraction is a reliable and ubiquitous measure of sexual orientation, but what exactly does it mean for you to be sexually attracted to someone? It must mean more to you than a guy is physically good-looking or works out a lot. Does it mean he's "hot," which implies sexual undertones?
- How does a boy crush differ from a best buddy or the kinds of intense friendships that are common during childhood and adolescence? At what point do feelings become infatua-tions rather than merely friendliness? And what exactly is a bromance and how does it fit with romantic attraction?
- Do straight guys have boy crushes as well?
- Is genital contact a meaningful indicator of mostly hetero-sexuality, or is it something widespread among straight boys in general? If a boy enjoys the encounter and finds it pleasurable, is that sufficient to indicate he's not exclusively straight and thus in your corner? Can a straight guy have sex with you or romantically love you without giving up his straightness?
- Is the type of sexual activity you engage in important? Is to receive oral sex or to be the inserter in anal sex of greater significance than mutual masturbation, genital rubbing, or genital displays? Are oral sex and anal intercourse equally meaningful?
- If you make out with another guy is it harmless and of little significance? Is French kissing of greater significance than lip

kissing? Can either be an indication of your romantic interest in a guy, separate from any desire to have sex with him or to entice women to be interested in you?

- Is developing or desiring a romantic relationship with a guy possible if you are a mostly straight guy, without stepping over the line into bisexuality?
- Are the characteristics reported here only true for your millennial generation or do they hold for older generations, despite their ability to suppress their sexual and romantic desires?
- What are the personality characteristics, situational variables, and cultural factors that influence stability and change in your sexual and romantic fluidity? Are curiosity and impulsiveness critical factors?
- What exactly is sexual and romantic fluidity anyway?

As we learn more about the lives of mostly straight young men, I look forward to hearing the answers.

escaping the sexual neverlands

You just never know. (DILLON, AGE 20)

GRANTED THAT SOME LIFE NARRATIVES in this book are likely to be more compelling to you than others. Perhaps it is the sexually oriented rather than the romantically oriented mostly straight young men who are more believable, or the reverse. Or it is the young men who supplied both romantic and sexual evidence as to their mostly straightness. I know Dillon was my breakpoint guy. After his story, I had to believe in mostly straight guys. That was all the testimony I needed—and you, too, I hope.

As you and additional young men of your generation recognize and reveal to others your sexual and romantic breadth and fluidity, you help the rest of us to understand the complexity of our sexual and romantic selves. Whether you are the new, gentle, emotionally sensitive young man or the masculine stud, when you admit to being "a little bit" attracted to a particular man and state that it's okay to act "gayish," you can help other teens and young men who have these feelings and are clamoring to *come out* as mostly straight. They, too, deserve to be released from their heterosexual straightjackets. We'll know that change has truly taken hold in our society when 13-year-old boys who are best buddies, spend all their time together, draw hearts with their names in them, sexually explore their bodies, and profess their friendship and love forever are deemed *normal*.

Unfortunately, many of you will remain closeted until as a society we conquer the stigma of same-sex sexuality, rejecting the disgust some feel when thinking about two guys in love or having sex. Given that *mostly straight* is the fastest growing sexual orientation identity today, who knows how many sexually and romantically fluid young men there are? Any current count is likely to underestimate the total.

Last year I did a workshop on mostly straights, and before the formal presentation I asked the forty youths to describe their sexual identity on a notecard. A 16-year-old boy wrote, "Straight, somewhat curious?" A 15-year-old was more elaborate: "Straitish, I suppose. I tend not to care, and I like who I like and love who I love, and while that's usually towards females, I can find men attractive, too. I don't know. I'm just me, and people are people." However, my favorite was a perfect lead-in to my talk, a 16-year-old boy who wrote, "I'd describe myself as Josh Hutcherson."

If more young men were to come out of the closet as mostly straight, we might better understand these dynamics, what promotes stability, and what furthers movement and fluctuation within the fluidity of individual lives—and answer the previous questions. My biggest hope, however, is that you'll see the merits of being open about your romantic and sexual self so that future generations of mostly straight boys and youths will understand and celebrate their straightness, with a twist.

Dillon, Josh, and the other young men you've just met here might show us the way. As Dillon inspired me, so may the young men enlighten all of us. Dillon did not emigrate or relinquish his sexual and romantic status during young adulthood. He has remained mostly straight. Starting now, let's purge young men from the murky landscape of the *sexual neverlands,* the invisible land that once existed between heterosexuality and bisexuality.

APPENDIXES

NOTES

ACKNOWLEDGMENTS

INDEX

APPENDIX A: methods

Among the young men I interviewed, eleven identified as straight with a slight degree of same-sex sexuality (primarily straight) and twenty-nine as mostly straight. They were participants in one of two research projects. In all respects, the protocol followed the ethical guidelines mandated by Cornell University where I was employed.

Friends and Lovers

From April 2008 through April 2009, 160 young men across a range of sexualities between the ages of 17 and 27 years (mean=20.0) volunteered for my Friends and Lovers study. The research was advertised as an interview study with young men about their "friends and lovers since you were a child, teenager, and now." By answering our questions, they would help us to increase our understanding regarding the sexual development of young men of all sexual orientations from earliest memories to the present time.

Seventy percent identified as Caucasian, with the rest identifying as Asian American (13 percent), African American (7 percent), Latino (6 percent), or Native American (3 percent). Of these young men, 72 percent were university students, and the remainder was enrolled in a local community or commuter college or was working. Their academic majors were widely distributed across the social sciences, biological/life sciences, engineering, and humanities. The most desired career trajectories were, in order, finance, marketing, or business; teaching (school teacher or professor); medicine (medical doctor or in the medical field); law; or engineering. Nearly three-quarters reported they were either middle or upper middle class. Two in ten reported that their families were working class or lower middle class. Two-thirds were raised in a small or medium-sized town or suburb, or a small city. Nearly one-third grew up in an urban area, and a few were from rural/farming communities.

Our flyers were posted in freshman and sophomore residence halls and college cafés. We also posted in online newsletters and on a fraternity email list. Our advertisement cards were hand-distributed by undergraduate research assistants, and participants also gave the advertisement cards to their friends. The young men who wished to participate notified me directly, as the primary investigator. The participants were then sent details regarding the project's purpose. If they wanted to participate, they were required to complete an informed consent form and were provided with a list of interview times. Once the interviews were scheduled, the participants were sent a preinterview survey requesting their basic demographic data (age, education, major, citizenship, ethnicity, social class, community size, and career objectives) and their high school and college activities, clubs, and organizations. They were informed that they should bring a completed hard copy with them to the interview.

The interview was held in a private location in an academic building on campus and lasted from 40 to 135 minutes, with an average of 73 minutes. At the beginning of the interview, each participant completed a questionnaire about what percentage of his sexual attractions, sexual interactions (genital contact), infatuations/crushes, sexual fantasies, and romantic relationships was directed to males and females when he was a child, an early adolescent, an adolescent, and now, and how he anticipates he will be and would like to be in the future. The interviews were not recorded, so the brief quotes provided throughout this book (usually with the generic "a young man") are not literally verbatim—but they are extremely close. I took extensive notes with a shorthand technique I've developed to record nearly every word, and I transcribed these notes immediately after each interview.

Eight individuals who volunteered for the study did not respond to further email contact to set up an interview time. Thus, 93 percent of the young men who contacted me completed the research. Of the participants who were sent a questionnaire, 100 percent returned it and 100 percent of those who set up an appointment completed the interview. Three did not show at the appointed time but contacted me and rescheduled.

The participants were paid a twenty-dollar incentive for their time. All but one agreed to be contacted in succeeding years to participate in longitudinal follow-up questionnaires, interviews, or experiments.

Of the 160 young men, nine were classified as primarily straight, and twenty identified as mostly straight. Of these 29 young men, the following (pseudonyms) are featured in this book: Chris as primarily straight, and Carlos, Dillon, Felix, Holland, Kevin, Luke, Mike, Sam, and Will as mostly straight young men. The others provided comments that are frequently included in the text.

Personality and Sexuality

Dr. Gerulf Rieger, a postdoctoral fellow in my Sex and Gender Lab, and his undergraduate research assistants recruited 229 participants in 2012. Of these, 109 were men between the ages of 18 and 32 (mean: 21.9). The research was broadly advertised as a lab-based study investigating issues of sex, gender, and personality. The primary purpose was the assessment of sexual orientation through a new technique, pupil dilation.

At the time, 66 percent of the men were undergraduate college students, and an additional 17 percent had completed their undergraduate education and were working. Others were in graduate school (9 percent), had completed some college and dropped out (6 percent), or had just finished high school (2 percent). Seventy-five percent identified as Caucasian and the rest as Asia American (12 percent), Latino (5 percent), mixed ethnicity/race (5 percent), and African American (4 percent).

Advertisements for the study were placed on a Facebook page, posted in several residence halls and fraternities, and posted on several websites that cater to members of athletic teams. To increase recruitment of sexual minorities, the study notice was also posted on a Craigslist forum oriented toward sexual minorities. Young men contacted the lab by email, and written informed consent was obtained once they arrived at the university lab. After they participated in the physiological portion of the study, they completed a survey administered online using an Internet-based survey tool, which included a 7-point sexual orientation scale identity, ranging from exclusively straight to exclusively gay. After they had completed the survey, I asked about their willingness to participate in an hour-long interview to "track your sexual and romantic development from first memories to the present day." All but four agreed to be contacted.

Of these 109 men, forty-six scheduled a follow-up interview for an additional incentive of twenty dollars. Of this group, two qualified as primarily straight (Demetri and Ricky) and nine as mostly straight (including Ben, Chandler, Jay, Joel, Kyle, and Ryan). All the names used in this book are pseudonyms. Informed consent was obtained to record these interviews, and a paid research assistant transcribed the recordings, which are the source of the quotes used in this book. The quotes have been altered only to mask personal identifying details and to delete extraneous information (e.g., a rant against a political party, an analysis of a participant's mother).

Reflections on Methods

These young men may or may not look like America in their basic personal and social lives, but it is not my intent to present them as representing anything other than themselves. They are diverse in many respects (social class, personality, religion, ethnicity, region), but I would never argue that they are "representative" of young men in the United States. Ideally, I wish more Latino, African American, and Native American young men had volunteered, that more young men who grew up in large urban areas with fewer socioeconomic resources had responded to the notices, that more young men of limited education (e.g., who never went to college) had felt comfortable participating in the research, and that more of the young men who were resistant to sharing their personal lives with a stranger had done so anyway.

Nearly a decade ago researchers Thompson and Morgan highlighted the uniqueness of mostly straight young women, bringing to our attention the need to "recognize and examine mostly straights as a distinct sexual identity subtype in young women." I agree. However, they did not give the same recognition to men, lumping mostly straight-identified college men in with bisexual and gay men as sexual minorities and contrasting them with heterosexual men, including a subset who questioned aspects of their sexuality. They concluded, "The standardized heterosexual identity appears simplistic." I agree. Unfortunately, they did not sufficiently believe that mostly straight men exist to give them a location on a sexual/romantic continuum.

Zhana Vrangalova, a graduate student, and I reviewed the scientific literature on mostly straight women *and* men, locating scores of studies. Here is an abbreviated and updated version for mostly straight men. We found five kinds of evidence to support the existence of mostly heterosexuality as a distinct sexuality.

1. Mostly straight has a unique sexual/romantic profile.
2. Mostly straight men have a distinguishing *physiological arousal pattern.*
3. A *significant number* of individuals identify as mostly straight.
4. The identification as mostly straight is fairly *stable* over time.
5. Mostly heterosexuality has *subjective relevance* for young men.

The last item is the essence of this book, beginning with the chapter "It Is Who I Am."

Profiling

A mostly straight youth exhibits sexual patterns of attraction, fantasy, and behavior and/or romantic patterns of infatuation and romance unique from straight men and bisexual men, his two adjacent neighbors along a sexual/romantic continuum. To be clear, in his sexual and romantic life he appears considerably closer to the straight guy than the bisexual guy.

If he were midway between the two you'd expect an ordered decrease in other-sex indicators and an ordered increase in same-sex indicators as you moved from heterosexuality to primarily heterosexuality, to mostly heterosexuality, and to bisexuality. This is *not* the case. In his sexual and romantic patterns, he is far more similar to straights and not merely intermediary or halfway between straight and bisexual men. For example, a typical straight man is 0 percent sexually attracted to men, a typical mostly straight man is 10 percent sexually attracted to men, and a typical bisexual man is 50 percent sexually attracted to men. And, equally important, a mostly straight man varies little from straight men in his sexual attraction to women—nearly 100 percent. How can he do this? A mostly straight man often says that his sexual attraction to men does not reduce his sexual attraction to women. Same-sex attraction is an addition, not a subtraction or a substitution. I have rarely found bisexual men who exhibit this pattern. Instead, they maintain substantial sexual attraction to both sexes, whether it is 30 percent/70 percent, 40 percent/60 percent, or 50 percent/50 percent.

In terms of sex, just to state the obvious, the vast majority of sex partners for both straight and mostly straight youths are female. This is less likely to be true for bisexual young men. However, what is nearly universal for all three is that they desire to have and have had sex with at least one woman. And, as you might expect, mostly straight men are more likely than straight men to have sex with another guy and less likely—and, if so, less frequently—than bisexual men to have male sex partners. For example, among British Columbia high school students who were sexually active during the past year, 6 percent of mostly straight boys had at least one same-sex partner. Among straight boys, fewer than 2 percent had sex with another guy (these might well be "primarily straight" boys), and among bisexual boys, nearly 50 percent had a same-sex partner. Again, mostly straight boys were considerably closer to straight than bisexual boys regarding the number who have had sex with another guy.

This pattern held not only for adolescents and young adults in Canada but also in Native American Indian nations, Alaska Native nations, Norway, the United Kingdom, New Zealand, Australia, and U.S. Facebook users.

What is not clear is whether the type of same-sex sexual behavior that mostly straight youths engage in differs from bisexual youths. Perhaps the sex a mostly straight youth has with men is more likely to be genital touching or mutual masturbation than oral or anal sex, or he is more likely to be the recipient than the giver of oral sex or the inserter than the recipient in anal intercourse. I believe this would be important information to know, but we don't. However, the young men I interviewed offered several clues about this issue: anal intercourse is off-limits, and the other guy frequently initiates the sexual contact.

Similar data on the romantic side (infatuation, romance) are not available, largely because researchers seldom collect such data. One small study indicated that mostly straight young men were far more likely than straight young men to report infatuations with other guys, though few of these evolved into dating or romantic relationships. This is in stark contrast to bisexual youths who frequently date and develop relationships with same-sex partners. My best guess is that on the romantic side, mostly straight youths duplicate the pattern they have with sexual attraction and behavior—more romantic feelings toward guys than straight men and considerably fewer than bisexual men.

Regardless, based on self-reports, mostly straight young men are unique from straight and bisexual men in their sexual and romantic profiles. They are not halfway between straight and bisexual young men, as they are far more straight than bisexual.

Genitals and Eyes Agree

Another method to assess the uniqueness of a mostly straight man is to rely not on his self-report of sexuality but to directly assess his physiological arousal to women and men. Involuntary measures of sexual orientation are relatively free of conscious control, which means any attempt he makes to present himself in a positive sexual light, however he defines it, would fail. There remains, as we would all likely agree, social stigma among some young men to having any degree of gayness, and if some of those men believe that they are mostly straight, they might not admit to having same-sex sexual or romantic attractions—or the desire to engage in sexual or romantic encounters with another man.

The most common way to measure physiological arousal is to assess penile enlargement (erection) to sexual stimuli. Recently, not only brain imaging but also determining pupil dilation (big eyes) to pornographic images has been added as an assessment tool. These arousal measures have their own limitations—they are time consuming, require a lab setup, are expensive, can include only a limited number of participants or sexual images on the screen, and are invasive, such as requiring a youth to place a band around the base of his penis to assess penile enlargement. However, physiological measures tap into processes that an individual himself might not know because his same-sex sexuality is so slight that he assumes it is normative for straight guys, or, as I mentioned before, he shares the stigma associated with responding positively to nude male images. Thus, physiological measures complement without replacing self-report measures of sexual and romantic orientations.

In my Sex and Gender Lab, Gerulf Rieger and others assessed both genital and pupil arousal to pornographic images of men and women masturbating. Mostly straight men responded to female stimuli exactly as straight men do, with an enlargement of the penis and eye pupils. However, they were more aroused by male stimuli than straight men but less so than bisexual men. The mostly straight man is not lying about his mostly straightness. He does not differ from a straight man in his enhanced physiological response to females but does in his heightened arousal to males. He also differs from a bisexual man in his higher response to females and lower response to males, as you might expect.

Prevalence

Another critical piece of evidence for the existence of mostly heterosexuality is the presence of a significant number of men in the general population who so identify. Across multiple studies, the prevalence rate of mostly heterosexuality among males varies considerably, usually ranging from as few as 2 percent to as many as 9 percent of the population. Among college students, the prevalence rate is slightly above average, about 7 percent. For example, national statistics out early in 2016 reported that 6 percent of young men between the ages of 18 and 24 claimed sexual attractions that are "mostly to the opposite sex," which was greater than any other age group.

Whether in fact fewer men than women are sexually fluid in that they have a slight degree of same-sex sexuality is uncertain. We only know that fewer men than women report it. Perhaps men fail to recognize that their feelings for other guys differ from other straight guys or that these desires say something meaningful about their sexual or romantic self. There is also still a prevailing social stigma of declaring any degree of same-sex sexuality. Taken together, these three factors likely deplete or at least silence the number of young men willing to identify as mostly straight. That is, although I can't tell you how many mostly straight young men remain unaware or closeted and are thus uncounted, my guess is that the current declaration of how many mostly straight guys there are in the population is likely an undercount rather than an overcount. What I can say with more confidence is that aside from exclusive heterosexuality, mostly heterosexuality is the largest point along the male sexual continuum, greater than bisexuality and homosexuality combined.

Developmentally, prevalence rates vary depending on the age of the individual. It is low during early and middle adolescence, high from late adolescence through early adulthood, and low again during older adulthood. The first contrast appears to be developmental. An adolescent boy might not yet recognize that his slight degree of same-sex sexuality is meaningful or unusual. As his homoeroticism persists throughout adolescence and as he enters young adulthood, he discovers others in his dorm, classes, or work environment who experience a similar degree of same-sex attraction and who have attached a name to it. Eventually his awareness increases, and he says, "Me, too."

The second contrast is likely a cohort effect, as the 2016 data indicate. It is not because of age but because of the time we live in. Youth of the millennial generation have greater levels of sexual knowledge, freedom, and exploration than do older generations. Older adults are less likely to label themselves as mostly straight because they don't know what it is. None of their friends identified as mostly straight. The true test of whether this is an age or cohort effect will be determined by whether the current generation of young men's reports of mostly straightness change with age, and whether generations coming after them take to mostly straightness in record numbers. I predict the latter will happen, largely because mostly straightness is a function both of developmental awareness of the meaning that a slight degree of same-sex romantic and sexual desires has and of social progress in terms of ensuing generations increasingly embracing sexual diversity and the sexual/romantic continuum.

Stability

Because sexual and romantic orientations are enduring, persistent characteristics of individuals regardless of their sexuality, stability is a fourth critical criterion for establishing the existence of mostly heterosexuality. If a mostly straight man's self-perception of his sexuality is persistent over time, rather than a result of a transitional state or a mistake, then this would support his genuine sexual and romantic point on the continuum.

Although most research indicates that a mostly straight identity is less stable over time than a straight identity, it is nevertheless more constant than a bisexual identity. As best as we can determine, about half of mostly straights maintain that identity, although we're not sure for how long because most studies have only short-term follow-up evaluations. In turn, of the few changes in sexual identity that occur among straight men, over 75 percent are toward mostly heterosexuality.

This latter finding reflects and reinforces the close kinship between exclusive straightness and mostly straightness. In a national sample of young men whose average age was 22, the proportion identifying as mostly straight slightly increased when they completed the same survey six years later. Tracking these changes reveals that when young men joined the ranks of mostly heterosexuals, they overwhelmingly came from the exclusively straight contingent and were not emigrants from the bisexual or gay categories (that is, guys going back into the closet). Similarly, if over time young men relinquished their mostly straight identity, over 80 percent turned to heterosexuality, not bisexuality or homosexuality. Thus, relatively few young men identified as mostly straight on their way to coming out as bisexual or gay. Rather, they re-upped their commitment to heterosexuality. Will they re-emerge as mostly straight later in life? We don't know yet.

Although developmental data regarding temporal stability of all sexualities are limited, they suggest that a mostly straight identification grows in stability from early adolescence through young adulthood. This is not surprising because adolescence is a time to explore the meaning of sexual and romantic feelings and is often followed by a corresponding increase in sexual identity consolidation as individuals move into adulthood.

Personal Meaningfulness

The fifth kind of evidence that supports the existence of mostly heterosexuality as a distinct sexuality is its meaningfulness in the lives of young men. The life histories that you have just read of young men who identify as mostly straight corroborate the unique integrity of mostly straightness.

Becoming Mostly Straight

If mostly heterosexuality is a true sexual and romantic orientation, it should be rooted in the same biological and environmental (prenatal) factors that determine all sexual orientations. As far as I can tell, no scientist is currently even considering investigating what causes men to be mostly heterosexual—so it may be some time before we definitely know its origins. In the meantime, my best bet is that the causes are consistent with the theories and research on sexual orientation origins, including by way of multiple genes or prenatal hormones that affect the neurological and endocrine systems that influence the direction of a boy's sexuality to erotic or romantic desires toward girls, boys, or both, to varying degrees. The key phrase here, as you are now well aware, is "to varying degrees."

From an evolutionary scenario, the prevailing view holds that men should be heterosexual and have procreative sex with women. Yet in order to maintain the species it is also possible to speculate that same-sex sexuality also benefits our species, whether it is extreme (gays) or partial (mostly straights, bisexuals). It is not difficult to imagine a scenario in which mostly heterosexuality was an evolutionary advantage—and perhaps a preferred one at that. For example, the extra dosage of male-loving genes or prenatal hormones might have increased a mostly straight man's sex appeal to females—given him greater sensitivity, more caring, less brutality, and greater child investment—and hence increased his desirability as a mate. More offspring reaching reproductive age may have been an outcome. In addition, the presence of some male-loving genes or hormones could have led to greater bonding with other men, resulting in mutual protection and sharing of resources during hunter/gatherer days. The result would be more protein, longer longevity, more offspring, and a greater input of genes into future generations—including whatever is responsible for determining a slight degree of same-sex sexuality.

Another route to mostly heterosexuality might be through a prenatal neuroendocrine process occurring during pregnancy that disrupts a male fetus from becoming totally attracted to females and becoming slightly attracted to males. Whatever it was would need to be sufficiently pervasive to alter the early brain development responsible for sexual and romantic determination. Possible causal agents for this biochemical event have been proposed, including maternal stress, drug/alcohol intake, or illness, and the mother's autoimmune response to "foreign" male fetal cells. Whatever the impact on the neuroendocrine system, the agent would not be so severe as to create complete same-sex sexuality but sufficient to produce a slightly altered heterosexual boy.

Consider one situation in which some boys may become gay: the fraternal birth order effect. With each pregnancy, some small number of fetal cells enters the mother's circulation. If the fetus is male, her immune system recognizes these male-specific molecules as *foreign* (that is, not female like herself) and in response produces antibodies to fight them. With each succeeding male fetus the antibody response becomes stronger, such that the likelihood of a totally gay son increases. Perhaps mostly straight sons are created through this same process. One way to test this would be to check whether mostly straight boys have a slight surplus of older brothers or, more telling, an excess of younger bisexual or gay brothers.

In brief, mostly straight men across developmental ages and cohorts report distinctive sexual and romantic profiles in terms of sexual arousal, attractions, fantasies, infatuations, behavior, and relationships. They are more same-sex oriented than straights, but less so than bisexuals. Physiological evidence confirms this uniqueness. Mostly straights constitute the largest nonheterosexual group, more numerous than all other nonheterosexual groups combined. A mostly heterosexual orientation is relatively stable over time; this stability is lower than for straights but typically higher than for bisexuals. Finally, those who identify as mostly straight testify to its subjective relevance. They indicate that they experience a small degree of sexual and romantic attractions to their nonpreferred sex.

By contrast, there's little evidence for alternative possibilities that a mostly heterosexual self-assessment is a result of nonsexual factors. For example, you might believe that a man who champions a mostly straight label is using it as a transitional identity, as an attempt to mask his "true" sexual orientation as bisexual or gay, or to acknowledge his (nonsexual) appreciation of male beauty, or as an expression of his political beliefs. Although these are valid reasons for some men, they're not prevalent and can be discounted by several findings.

First, almost no mostly straight man said he chose a bisexual/gay identity when a mostly heterosexual one was not available. Second, few men changed from a mostly straight identity in the direction of a bisexual or gay identity. Third, the pro-gay affiliation that many mostly straight young men espoused and their generally progressive sexual attitudes do not support the speculation that they are hiding from the stigma of homosexuality.

However, this last led me to further wonder if they were identifying as not totally straight for political reasons or to be edgy or provocative. This is a worthy consideration but one that was minimized by the young men in this book who narrated their sexual and romantic lives.

Young people today explicitly tell us that any measure of their sexuality that does not provide a mostly straight option is incompetence. It is an unfair and a misguided attempt to limit a genuine, accurate accounting of sexuality. If it's not presented as a possibility, he'll be forced to select something he is not (exclusively straight) or just leave the question blank. Or he might check "other," which is vague and difficult to decipher for those of us on the outside. Rather, we should listen to him when he tells us about himself.

notes

Preface

For definitions of millennial, in terms of years born and unique characteristics, see the Urban Dictionary at www.urbandictionary.com. Although the dates may vary, the millennial generation was born between the mid-1980s and the turn of the century.

For questions and data regarding the survey, see Peter Moore, "A Third of Young Americans Say They Aren't 100% Heterosexual," YouGov, August 20, 2015, https://today.yougov.com/news/2015/08/20/third-young-americans-exclusively -heterosexual. The same age trends reported in the U.S. survey also characterized those from the United Kingdom and Israel, and likely many other people worldwide.

For information on the women's literature, see R. C. Savin-Williams and Z. Vrangalova, "Mostly Heterosexual as a Distinct Sexual Orientation Group: A Systematic Review of the Empirical Evidence," *Developmental Review* 33 (2013): 58–88.

Polling data are available from the Pew Research Report, which is discussed in Sam Tanenhaus, "Generation Nice: The Millennials Are Generation Nice," *New York Times*, August 15, 2014, www.nytimes.com/2014/08/17 /fashion/the-millennials-are-generation-nice.html. Also see J. M. Twenge, R. A. Sherman, and S. Lyubomirsky, "More Happiness for Young People and Less for Mature Adults: Time Period Differences in Subjective Well-Being in the United States, 1972–2014," *Social Psychological and Personality Science* 7 (2016): 131–141; and J. M. Twenge, R. A. Sherman, and B. E. Wells, "Changes in American Adults' Sexual Behavior and Attitudes," *Archives of Sexual Behavior* 44 (2015): 2273–2285. Polling data on the millennial generation also are available online from the nonprofit Public Religion Research Institute (PRRI), led R. P. Jones and D. Cox, at www.publicreligion.org.

Dillon is featured in an online magazine article: R. C. Savin-Williams and K. M. Cohen, "Mostly Straight, Most of the Time," *The Good Men Project*, November 3, 2010, http://goodmenproject.com/2010/11/03/mostly-straight/.

The Sexual Neverlands

For recent prevalence rates, see C. E. Copen, A. Chandra, and I. Febo-Vazquez, "Sexual Behavior, Sexual Attraction, and Sexual Orientation among Adults Aged 18–44 in the United States: Data from the 2011–2013 National Survey of Family Growth," *National Health Statistics Reports*, no. 88 (Washington, DC: U.S. Department of Health and Human Services, January 2016).

Straight but Not Narrow

Information about Straight But Not Narrow can be found at www.straight butnotnarrow.org. For an interview with Josh Hutcherson, see Shana Naomi Krochmal, "Josh Hutcherson, Straight Talker," *Out*, October 9, 2013, www.out .com/entertainment/movies/2013/10/09/josh-hutcherson-straight-talker-hunger -games-threesome.

Ezra Miller's interviews can be found at two locations: Jeremy Kinser, "Ezra Miller: *Perks of Being a Wallflower* Star Comes Out," *The Advocate*, August 15, 2012, www.advocate.com/arts-entertainment/film/2012/08/15/ezra-miller-perks -being-wallflower-star-comes-out; and Marlow Stern, "Ezra Miller on 'Perks of Being a Wallflower,' Being Bisexual & More," *Daily Beast*, September 18, 2012, www.thedailybeast.com/articles/2012/09/18/ezra-miller-on-perks-of-being-a -wallflower-being-bisexual-more.html.

Freddy Fox's interview is at "Freddie Fox Suggests He Is Bisexual as He Says He Could 'Fall in Love with a Man,' " *Daily Telegraph* [UK], January 18, 2015, www.telegraph.co.uk/news/celebritynews/11354179/Freddie-Fox-suggests -he-is-bisexual-as-he-says-he-could-fall-in-love-with-a-man.html.

Jack Falahee's interview is at Curtis M. Wong, " 'How to Get Away with Murder' Star Jack Falahee Won't Reveal His Sexuality Because It 'Feels Reductive,' " *Huffington Post*, February 11, 2015, www.huffingtonpost.com/2015/02 /11/jack-falahee-sexuality-_n_6661016.html.

Jake Uitti published his story last year: Jack Uitti, "I'm in My 30s. Is It Too Late to Explore My Sexuality?," *Washington Post*, July 15, 2016, www .washingtonpost.com/news/soloish/wp/2016/07/15/im-in-my-30s-is-it-too-late-to -explore-my-sexuality.

Again, Dillon's story was originally chronicled at R. C. Savin-Williams and K. M. Cohen, "Mostly Straight, Most of the Time," *The Good Men Project*, November 3, 2010, http://goodmenproject.com/2010/11/03/mostly-straight/.

Sexual and Romantic Spectrums

For the Kinsey research, see A. C. Kinsey, W. B. Pomeroy, and C. E. Martin, *Sexual Behavior in the Human Male* (Philadelphia: W. B. Saunders, 1948).

For further discussion of the category versus continuum approaches, see R. C. Savin-Williams, "Sexual Orientation: Categories or Continuum? Commentary on Bailey et al. (2016)," *Psychological Science in the Public Interest* 17 (2016): 37–44; and R. C. Savin-Williams, "An Exploratory Study of the Categorical versus Spectrum Nature of Sexual Orientation," *Journal of Sex Research* 51 (2014): 446–453. The primary advocates for the lumpers have been J. M. Bailey, P. L. Vasey, L. D. Diamond, S. M. Breedlove, E. Vilain, and M. Epprecht, "Sexual Orientation, Controversy, and Science," *Psychological Science in the Public Interest* 17 (2016): 45–101; and J. M. Bailey, "What Is Sexual Orientation and Do Women Have One?," in *Contemporary Perspectives on Lesbian, Gay, and Bisexual Identities*, vol. 54, ed. D. A. Hope, 43–63 (New York: Springer, 2009). For discussion of the lumpers and the splitters, see J. D. Weinrich, P. J. Snyder, R. C. Pillard, I. Grant, D. L. Jacobson, S. Renée Robinson, and J. A. McCutchan, "A Factor Analysis of the Klein Sexual Orientation Grid in Two Disparate Samples," *Archives of Sexual Behavior* 22 (1993): 157–168.

Romantic Orientation

Several early sex scholars, such as Kinsey, included a psychological component, an *affectional disposition*, or an emotional preference to their sexual orientation measure. For Kinsey's research, see A. C. Kinsey, W. B. Pomeroy, and C. E. Martin, *Sexual Behavior in the Human Male* (Philadelphia: W. B. Saunders, 1948). Other early measures and research include J. C. Gonsiorek, R. L. Sell, and J. D. Weinrich, "Definition and Measurement of Sexual Orientation," *Suicide and Life-Threatening Behavior* 25, no. S1 (1995): 40–51; F. Klein, B. Sepekoff, and T. J. Wolf, "Sexual Orientation: A Multi-variable Dynamic Process," *Journal of Homosexuality* 11 (1985): 35–49; R. L. Sell, "The Sell Assessment of Sexual Orientation: Background and Scoring," *Journal of Gay, Lesbian, and Bisexual Identity* 1 (1996): 295–310; M. G. Shively and J. P. DeCecco, "Components of Sexual Identity," *Journal of Homosexuality* 3 (1977): 41–48; and J. D. Weinrich, P. J. Snyder, R. C. Pillard, I. Grant, D. L. Jacobson, S. R. Robinson, and J. A. McCutchan, "A Factor Analysis of the Klein Sexual Orientation Grid in Two Disparate Samples," *Archives of Sexual Behavior* 22 (1993): 157–168.

Romantic references are located at R. J. Sternberg, "Triangulating Love," in *The Psychology of Love*, ed. R. J. Sternberg and M. L. Barnes, 119–138 (New Haven, CT: Yale University Press, 1988); E. Hatfield and R. L. Rapson, "Passionate Love/Sexual Desire: Can the Same Paradigm Explain Both?," *Archives of Sexual Behavior* 16 (1987): 259–278; E. Hatfield and R. L. Rapson, "The Neuropsychology of Passionate Love," in *Psychology of Relationships*, ed. E. Cuyler and M. Ackhart, 519–543 (Hauppauge, NY: Nova Science Publishers, 2009); V. Karandashev and S. Clapp, "Psychometric Properties and Structures of Passionate and Companionate Love," *Interpersona* 10 (2016): 56–76; and H. E. Fisher, *Why We Love: The Nature and Chemistry of Romantic Love* (New York: Henry Holt, 2004).

Adolescents' views about sexual orientation are provided in M. S. Friedman, A. J. Silvestre, M. A. Gold, N. Markovic, R. C. Savin-Williams, J. Huggins, and R. L. Sell, "Adolescents Define Sexual Orientation and Suggest Ways to Measure It," *Journal of Adolescence* 27 (2004): 303–317.

Sexual and Romantic Fluidity

For definitions of the various terms that have received publicity, primarily on social media, see the Urban Dictionary at www.urbandictionary.com.

Lisa Diamond defined fluidity in her lecture on October 17, 2013, to the Department of Human Development, Cornell University, Ithaca, NY. Also see her book *Sexual Fluidity: Understanding Women's Love and Desire* (Cambridge, MA: Harvard University Press, 2008).

Stories for each magazine can be found at Alexa Tsoulis-Reay, "Are You Straight, Gay, or Just . . . You?," *Glamour,* February 11, 2016, www.glamour.com /sex-love-life/2016/02/glamour-sexuality-survey; Eric Sasson, "Kristen Stewart, Miley Cyrus and the Rise of Sexual Fluidity," *Wall Street Journal,* August 17, 2015, http://blogs.wsj.com/speakeasy/2015/08/17/kristen-stewart-miley-cyrus-and -the-rise-of-sexual-fluidity; and Evan Urquhart, "What Do We Really Mean When We Say Women Are Sexually 'Fluid?,' " *Slate,* September 26, 2014, www.slate .com/blogs/outward/2014/09/26/why_the_sexual_fluidity_trope_is_sexism_in _disguise.html.

It Is Who I Am

Parts of this section are based on R. C. Savin-Williams, "The New Sexual-Minority Teenager: Freedom from Traditional Notions of Sexual Identity," in *The Meaning of Sexual Identity in the Twenty-first Century,* ed. Judith S. Kaufman and David A. Powell, 5–20 (Newcastle upon Tyne, UK: Cambridge Scholars, 2014).

Straight, but Not Totally Straight

Prevalence rates are reported in C. E. Copen, A. Chandra, and I. Febo-Vazquez, "Sexual Behavior, Sexual Attraction, and Sexual Orientation among Adults Aged 18–44 in the United States: Data from the 2011–2013 National Survey of Family Growth," *National Health Statistics Reports,* no. 88 (Washington, DC: U.S. Department of Health and Human Services, January 2016).

For research on gay sex among straight men, see A. M. Fasula, E. Oraka, W. L. Jeffries IV, M. Carry, M. C. Bañez Ocfemia, A. B. Balaji, C. E. Rose, and P. E. Jayne, "Young Sexual Minority Males in the United States: Sociodemographic Characteristics and Sexual Attraction, Identity and Behavior," *Perspectives on Reproductive and Sexual Health* 48 (2016): 3–8.

For a queer perspective, see Graham Gremore, "Straight Men Are a Lot More Bisexual Than You Might Think," *Queerty,* October 25, 2014, www.queerty .com/straight-men-are-a-lot-more-bisexual-than-people-think-20141025.

For a discussion of gay youths' attitudes toward other gay youths, see R. C. Savin-Williams, *Becoming Who I Am: Young Men on Being Gay* (Cambridge, MA: Harvard University Press, 2016).

Do Mostly Straight Youth Exist?

The names in the gay and mostly gay section are from an earlier book on the lives of gay young men: R. C. Savin-Williams, *Becoming Who I Am: Young Men on Being Gay* (Cambridge, MA: Harvard University Press, 2016).

Developmental Trajectories

This literature for this section is summarized in two of my previous books: R. C. Savin-Williams, *Becoming Who I Am: Young Men on Being Gay* (Cambridge, MA: Harvard University Press, 2016), and *The New Gay Teenager* (Cambridge, MA: Harvard University Press, 2005). Also see A. P. Smiler, *Dating and Sex: A Guide for the 21st Century Teen Boy* (Washington, DC: American Psychological Association, 2016).

The importance of self-esteem is found in D. Van de Bongardt, E. Reitz, and M. Dekovic, "Indirect Over-Time Relations between Parenting and Adolescents' Sexual Behaviors and Emotions through Global Self-esteem," *Journal of Sex Research* 53 (2016): 273–285.

A recent review of pornography is provided by J. Peter and P. M. Valkenburg, "Adolescents and Pornography: A Review of 20 Years of Research," *Journal of Sex Research* 53 (2016): 509–531.

Gaydar is reviewed in N. O. Rule and R. Alaei, "Gaydar: The Perception of Sexual Orientation from Subtle Cues," *Current Directions in Psychological Science* 25 (2016): 444–448, doi: 10.1177/0963721416664403.

If You Believe You Are Mostly Straight

For discussion of homohysteria, see M. McCormack, *The Declining Significance of Homophobia: How Teenage Boys Are Redefining Masculinity and Heterosexuality* (New York: Oxford University Press, 2012).

Appendix B: Mostly Straight Science

See E. Thompson and E. M. Morgan, "'Mostly Straight' Young Women: Variations in Sexual Behavior and Identity Development," *Developmental Psychology* 44 (2008): 15–21; and E. M. Morgan, M. G. Steiner, and E. M. Thompson, "Processes of Sexual Orientation Questioning among Heterosexual Men," *Men and Masculinities* 12 (2010): 425–443.

The review of the mostly straight developmental literature is found in R. C. Savin-Williams and Z. Vrangalova, "Mostly Heterosexual as a Distinct Sexual Orientation Group: A Systematic Review of the Empirical Evidence," *Developmental Review* 33 (2013): 58–88. (If you can't locate it, email me at Savin-Williams@cornell.edu.)

The Canadian study is C. S. Poon and E. M. Saewyc, "Out Yonder: Sexual-Minority Adolescents in Rural Communities in British Columbia," *American Journal of Public Health* 99 (2009): 118–124. For a review of the other countries, see Savin-Williams and Vrangalova, "Mostly Heterosexual."

The small study is R. C. Savin-Williams, "An Exploratory Study of the Categorical versus Spectrum Nature of Sexual Orientation," *Journal of Sex Research* 51 (2014): 446–453.

The physiological data are reported in research conducted by Gerulf Rieger in my Sex and Gender Lab: G. Rieger, B. M. Cash, S. M. Merrill, J. Jones-Rounds, S. Dharmavaram, and R. C. Savin-Williams, "Sexual Arousal: The Correspondence of Eyes and Genitals," *Biological Psychology* 104 (2015): 56–64; M. C. Stief, G. Rieger, and R. C. Savin-Williams, "Bisexuality Is Associated with Elevated Sexual Sensation Seeking, Sexual Curiosity, and Sexual Excitability," *Personality and Individual Differences* 66 (2014): 193–198; G. Rieger, A. M. Rosenthal, B. M. Cash, J. A. W. Linsenmeier, J. M. Bailey, and R. C. Savin-Williams, "Male Bisexual Arousal: A Matter of Curiosity?," *Biological Psychology* 94 (2013): 479–489; R. C. Savin-Williams, G. Rieger, and A. M. Rosenthal, "Physiological Evidence for a Mostly Heterosexual Orientation among Men," *Archives of Sexual Behavior* 42 (2013): 697–699; and G. Rieger and R. C. Savin-Williams, "The Eyes Have It: Sex and Sexual Orientation Differences in Pupil Dilation Patterns," *PLoS ONE* 7 (2012): e40256.

Prevalence rates are reported in C. E. Copen, A. Chandra, and I. Febo-Vazquez, "Sexual Behavior, Sexual Attraction, and Sexual Orientation among Adults Aged 18–44 in the United States: Data from the 2011–2013 National Survey of Family Growth," *National Health Statistics Reports,* no. 88 (Washington, DC: U.S. Department of Health and Human Services, January, 2016).

Stability data are available from the National Longitudinal Study of Adolescent to Adult Health: see R. C. Savin-Williams, K. Joyner, and G. Rieger, "Prevalence and Stability of Self-Reported Sexual Orientation Identity during Young Adulthood," *Archives of Sexual Behavior* 41 (2012): 103–110.

Blanchard's views are best expressed in R. Blanchard, "Quantitative and Theoretical Analyses of the Relation between Older Brothers and Homosexuality in Men," *Journal of Theoretical Biology* 230 (2004): 173–187.

acknowledgments

I would like to thank the young men, particularly those who are the foundation of this book, who are secure in their sexual and romantic selves to identify as mostly straight. My special thanks also goes out to actor Josh Hutcherson, a pioneer of this movement who shares with his millennial generation the possibility of being open, honest, revolutionary, and mostly straight.

This project might never have happened without the inspiration of one of the most delightful young men I have met, who must go by the pseudonym Dillon to comply with the ethical obligations of my university for confidentiality of research participants. Dillon's story was first told online in the *Good Men Project* magazine, thanks to the invitation of the editor, Benoit Denizet-Lewis. Little did I know after that first interview with Dillon that he and I would talk again and again, such that ten years later we have maintained contact as he approaches the magical age of 30.

Having worked with several publishers during my professional life, I am thrilled to continue with Harvard University Press because of the quality of its staff, the support HUP provides to authors, and the press's willingness to take risks with authors. My editor, Andrew Kinney, along with his extremely capable colleagues, Katrina Vassallo and Olivia Woods (editorial assistants), Andrew Martin (senior publicist), and Michael Higgins (marketing and promotions coordinator), followed the HUP tradition of excellence. They have been a pure delight to work with.

I am grateful to Fritz Klein (founder) and John Sylla (chairman and chief executive officer) of the American Institute of Bisexuality for financial support during the past four years. My home department, Human Development; college, Human Ecology; and university, Cornell, have been unyielding in their encouragement and support.

Finally, I am able to write because I have one of the most loving and supportive husbands in the universe, Kenneth Miles Cohen.

index

Alcohol, 97, 107, 152, 189, 220
Anal sex, 18, 35, 41, 79, 114, 132, 146, 189, 200, 202, 215
Anxiety, 12, 25–26, 124, 139–140, 181
Arousal, 11, 23, 29, 37, 105, 168, 177–178, 192, 196, 200, 215–216, 221
Asexuality, 64–65, 122, 154
Athletics/athletes, 3, 12, 14–15, 17, 35, 37–38, 40, 77, 82, 87, 95, 104, 110, 119–120, 182, 194, 211. *See also* Jocks; Sports
Attachment, 15–16, 26–27, 120, 123, 131, 135, 156, 158, 171, 177
Attitudes, 14, 19, 124, 148, 195–196; progressive, x, 19, 42, 72–73, 154, 221; toward gays, 39–41, 158, 177–178
Attractiveness, 7, 31, 36, 53–54, 62, 73, 77–78, 83, 88, 108, 115, 121, 123, 128, 154, 189–190, 198

Bars (gay), 17, 20, 169, 174
Bars (straight), 169, 172–173
Ben, 128–133, 136–137, 154, 212
"Bicurious," 1, 85, 90, 121–122, 161, 190
Bisexuality, 1, 5, 21, 23, 83, 102, 111, 136, 154–155, 193, 198, 203, 205, 214, 217, 219
Bisexual-leaning straight, ix, 23, 98, 165
Bisexual phase, vii, 165
Blow job, 34, 87–89, 117, 130, 136, 138, 145–146, 189. *See also* Oral sex
Boyfriends, vii, 86, 170, 173

Brothers, vii, 4, 53–55, 80, 84, 101, 104–105, 111–112, 163, 183–185, 221

Carlos, x, 115–119, 121–122, 211
Casual sex (females), x, 40, 98, 171. *See also* Hookups
Casual sex (males), 98. *See also* Hookups
Chandler, 128, 137, 212; interview, 147–148; childhood, 148–149; adolescence, 149–151; dating and sex, 151–152; sexual and romantic status, 152–154; musings, 154–155
Chris, 45, 211; interview, 66–67; childhood, 67–68; adolescence, 68–69; dating and sex, 69; sexual and romantic status, 70–71; musings, 71
Coming out (as mostly straight), 73, 75, 109, 154, 160, 165, 169, 171, 173, 180–181, 184, 200–201, 205, 219
Condoms, 16, 51, 58, 61, 69, 86, 88, 118, 126, 151, 185, 188. *See also* Safe sex
Confidence, x, 8, 44, 62, 67–68, 107, 131, 134, 154, 163, 183, 202, 217
Crush/infatuation, x, 3, 25–27, 114, 179, 192–195, 210, 213, 215, 221; on boys, 2–3, 20, 28–29, 34, 36, 39, 42–43, 52, 62–63, 66, 73, 83, 87, 91, 98–99, 107, 113–114, 118, 120, 123, 127, 129, 131, 133, 135–136, 138, 145–146, 152, 168, 171, 175–176, 178, 182, 190, 201–202, 215; on girls, 13, 46, 48, 54, 58, 63, 67, 81–82, 84, 86, 91, 94, 98,